LAB INTERPRETATION

The Indispensable Guide to Quickly Learn and Interpret The Laboratory Results. Find and Understand Everything That Impacts a Diagnosis of Disease.

Anne Jastinton

© **Copyright 2021 - All rights reserved.**

This document is geared towards providing exact and reliable information in regard to the topic and issue covered.

- From a Declaration of Principles which was accepted and approved equally by a Committee of the American Bar Association and a Committee of Publishers and Associations.

In no way is it legal to reproduce, duplicate, or transmit any part of this document in either electronic means or in printed format. All rights reserved.

The information provided herein is stated to be truthful and consistent, in that any liability, in terms of inattention or otherwise, by any usage or abuse of any policies, processes, or directions contained within is the solitary and utter responsibility of the recipient reader. Under no circumstances will any legal responsibility or blame be held against the publisher for any reparation, damages, or monetary loss due to the information herein, either directly or indirectly.

Respective authors own all copyrights not held by the publisher.

The information herein is offered for informational purposes solely and is universal as so. The presentation of the information is without contract or any type of guarantee assurance.

The trademarks that are used are without any consent, and the publication of the trademark is without permission or backing by the trademark owner. All trademarks and brands within this book are for clarifying purposes only and are owned by the owners themselves, not affiliated with this document.

Table of Contents

Chapter 1: Understanding Laboratory Values 11
    Benefit Vs. Risk Considerations of the Therapeutic Intervention 12
    What Do My Laboratory Results Mean? 13
    Chronic Vs. Acute Considerations of the Therapeutic Intervention. 15

Chapter 2: Correct Methods to Obtain Laboratory Samples 17
    Obtaining Dependable and Precise Laboratory Test Results 18
        1. Avoid mistakes in patient identification 18
        2. Draw the tubes in the correct order 18
        3. Use proper collecting containers 19
        4. Immediately after collection, gently invert all tubes 10 times .. 20
        5. Do not transfer specimens from one type of container to another 20
        6. Submit specimens to the laboratory as soon as possible 20
    For Specimens Collected Away from Campus 20
    Laboratory Specimen Storage Temperature Requirements 21
        1. Avoid hemolysis 21
        2. Drawing samples from a line 22
    Samples Eliminated from the Body Naturally 22
        Semen 23
        Sputum 23
        Stool 23
        Urine 24
        Saliva 25
        Oral fluid 25
        Sweat 25
    Simple-to-Obtain Specimens 25
        Examples 25
            Female reproductive system secretions and tissues 26
            Fluids and secretions from the nose or throat 26

      Open wounds and sores samples 26
      Other 27
   Samples from Within 27
      Examples 28
         Blood 28
         Tissue biopsy 28
         Needle biopsy 28
         An excisional biopsy 29
   Cerebrospinal Fluid (CSF) 29
   Additional Bodily Fluids 30
      Bone marrow 30
   Amniotic Fluid 31

Chapter 3: Hematological Tests 32
   Test: Total Hemoglobin (Hgb or Hb) 33
      Clinical implications 33
   Fetal Hemoglobin 33
   Hemoglobin Type and Distribution Variations (in Adults) 35
   Test: Hemoglobin Electrophoresis 35
   Test: Hematocrit (Hct) 37
      Clinical implications 37
   Test: Red Blood Cell Count (RBC count) 37
      Clinical implications 38
   Test: Red Cell Indices (Wintrobe Indices) 38
      1. MCV — Mean corpuscular volume 38
         Clinical implications 39
      2. MCH — Mean corpuscular hemoglobin 39
      3. MCHC — Mean corpuscular hemoglobin concentration 39
         Clinical implications 40
   Test: Reticulocyte Count (Retic count) 40
      Clinical implications 40
   Test: Sickle Cell Test 40

Test: Iron and Total Iron-Binding Capacity 41
Test: Ferritin 42
Test: ESR — Erythrocyte Sedimentation Rate 43
Test: Osmotic Fragility 45
Test: WBC Count — White Blood Cell Count (Leukocyte Count) 46
Basic Types of WBC 46
    Clinical implications 46
Test: Differential Cell Count Also Known as "Diff" or "Differential" 47
    Clinical implications 47
WBC Levels 48

Chapter 4: Serum Electrolytes Tests 49
Test: Sodium, (Na Serum) 52
    Clinical implications 52
Test: Potassium, (K+) 53
    Clinical implications 53
Test: Chloride, (Cl) 53
    Clinical implications 53
Test: Serum Osmolality 54
    Clinical implications 55
Test: Acid Phosphatase 55
    Clinical implications 56
Test: Ammonia Measures Plasma Levels of Ammonia 56
    Clinical implications 57
Test: Creatinine 58
    Clinical implications 58

Chapter 5: Test for Heart Disease 60
Symptoms of Heart Disease 60
Physical Exam and Blood Tests 61
Non-invasive Tests for Heart Disease 62
    Electrocardiogram 63
    Echocardiogram 63

 The stress test 63
 Carotid ultrasound 63
 Holter monitor 64
 Chest X-ray 64
 Tilt table test 64
 A CT scans 64
 MRI of the heart 65
Invasive Tests to Diagnose Heart Disease 65
 Coronary angiography and cardiac catheterization 65
 Electrophysiology study 65
 When to see your doctor 66
Common Medical Tests to Diagnose Heart Conditions 66
 Blood tests 67
 Electrocardiogram (ECG) 67
 Exercise stress test 67
 Echocardiogram (ultrasound) 68
 Nuclear cardiac stress test 68
 Coronary angiogram 68
 Magnetic resonance imaging (MRI) 69
 Coronary computed tomography angiogram (CCTA) 69
Blood Tests for Heart Disease 69
 Test: cholesterol 70
 High-sensitivity C-reactive protein 71
 Lipoprotein (a) 72
 Plasma ceramides 73
 Natriuretic peptides 73
 Troponin T 74
Chapter 6: Serological Tests for Specific Infections **75**
Serological Examinations 76
 Bacterial Infections 77
 Infections caused by viruses 78

Others 78
   1. Atypical primary pneumonia 78
   2. Rickettsial infections 78
   3. Mononucleosis infectious 79
   4. Mycotic infections 79
   5. Inflammatory conditions 79
   6. Rheumatoid arthritis 80
What Are the Different Types of Serology Tests and How Do They Work? 80
What Types of Serology Testing Are Available? 83
   Rapid serology test (RST) 83
   Enzyme-Linked immunosorbent assay (ELISA) 83
   Neutralization assay 83
   Chemiluminescent immunoassay 84
Serology Tests Are Classified into the Following Categories 85

Chapter 7: Tumor Markers 87
What Exactly Are Tumor Markers? 87
   Limitations 88
How are Tumor Markers Used? 89
   Assist in the diagnosis 89
   Stage 89
   Screen 90
   Assist with therapy selection 90
   Ascertain the prognosis 90
   Track treatment success and detect recurrence 90
Table of Tumor Marker Examples 91

Chapter 8: Testing for Body Fluid and Stool 100
What Exactly Are Off-Label Body Fluids? 101
   What are the difficulties of off-label body fluid testing? 101
   Is there off-label body fluid testing guidance available? 102
How Can Laboratories Lower Their Risk? 103

The Purpose and Practicality of Body Fluid Validation and Testing 104
The Role of Laboratories in Patient Management 105
Transforming Body Fluid Challenges into Lessons Learned 106
    Lesson 1 107
    Challenge 2 108
    Lesson 2 108
    Challenge 3 109
    Lesson 3 109
    Challenge 4 109
    Lesson 4 110

Chapter 9: Arterial Blood Gas Analysis 112

Blood Gas Test 114
Why Is a Blood Gas Test Performed? 115
What Are the Risks Associated with a Blood Gas Test? 116
    How does a blood gas test work? 116
Explaining The Result of a Blood Gas Test 117
    The test assesses: 118
        Arterial blood pH 118
        Bicarbonate 118
        Partial oxygen pressure 118
        Carbon dioxide partial pressure 118
        Oxygen saturation 118

Chapter 10: Renal Function Tests 120

Specimen Collection 121
Procedures 122
    Renal function assessment 122
    Glomerular filtration rate 122
    Creatinine 123
Blood Urea Nitrogen (BUN) 125
    BUN proportion 126
Cystatin C 126

    Albuminuria and proteinuria 127
        Glomerular proteinuria 127
        Tubular proteinuria 127
        Overflow proteinuria 128
        Irritation or tumor of the urinary tract 128
    Tubular Function Tests 128
    Urine Examination 129
    Acute Renal Impairment Vs. Chronic Renal Impairment 131
    Novel Biomarkers 133
        Indications 134
        Potential diagnosis 134
        Normal and critical finding 135
    Internal Factors 135
        Creatinine 135
        BUN 136
        Protein and urine albumin 136
        Complications 136
        Patient safety and awareness 136

Chapter 11: Liver Function Tests 138
    What Exactly Are Liver Function Tests? 138
    Which of the Following Are the Most Prevalent Liver Function Tests? 140
        Alanine transaminase (ALT) test 140
        Aspartate aminotransferase (AST) test 140
        Alkaline phosphatase (ALP) test 141
        Albumin test 141
        Bilirubin test 142
    What Is the Purpose of a Liver Function Test? 142
    What Are the Signs and Symptoms of a Liver Disease? 143
    Preparing for a Liver Function Test 143
        The Risks of a Liver Function Test 145

    After a liver function test 145

Chapter 12: Endocrine Function Test 147

    Endocrine Function Fertility Tests 148

        ACTH (adrenocorticotropic hormone) 148

        Aldosterone 148

        C-Peptide 148

        CA-125 149

        Cortisol 149

        Growth hormone 149

        Insulin 150

        T3 (Triiodothyronine) 150

        T4 (Thyroxine) 150

        TSH (Thyroid-stimulating hormone) 152

        Thyroid Peroxidase Antibody (TPO Ab) 152

        Vitamin D 25 OH 152

Chapter 13: Miscellaneous Diagnostic Tests 153

    Skin Prick Tests 153

    Aspects of Application 154

    Rast 155

    Unconventional Tests 155

    Induced Sputum Technique 155

    Bronchoprovocation Test 156

        Non-specific bronchoprovocation test 156

    Cardiac Enzymes Discussion 157

    Test: Myoglobin 158

        Clinical implications 159

Conclusion 160

Chapter 1: Understanding Laboratory Values

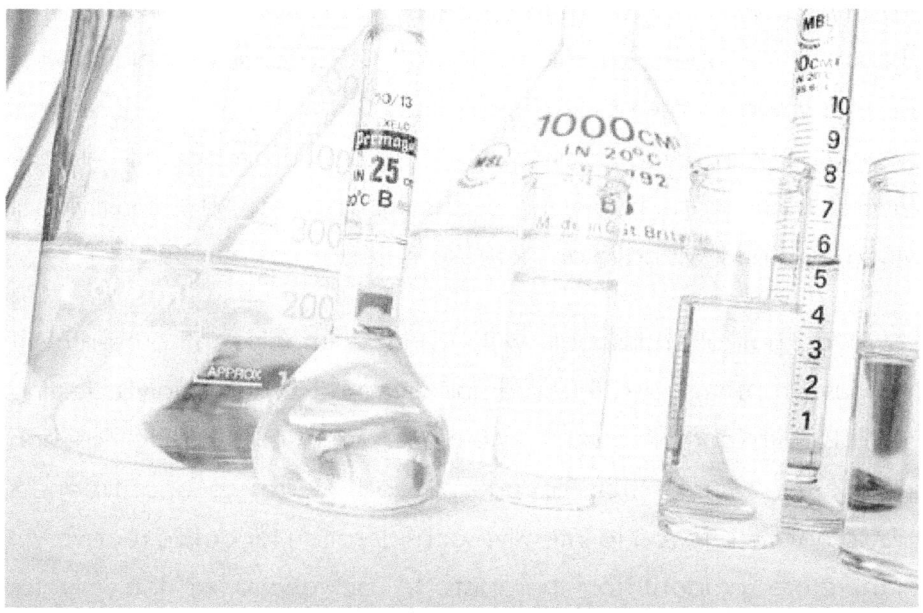

Physical therapists should not rely simply on a single laboratory report; rather, they should consider a variety of additional clinical factors. Clinicians, for example, should be aware of the time when laboratory test was collected, any drug interactions, and the patient's most recent meals. Similarly, it is critical to grasp the significance of patterns in values across time. Electrolyte panels may vary as a result of intravenous medicines, infusions, and dietary changes. Patients with chronic illnesses, such as anemia, may be asymptomatic during exercise, but a patient with a significant reduction in hematocrit and hemoglobin may require immediate medical attention.

When a patient arrives with symptoms of a suspected myocardial dead tissue (MI), cardiac biomarker laboratory tests are ordered to aid in the differential diagnosis. Cardiac biomarkers are substances released into the circulatory system when the heart is under stress or strain. In normal circumstances, these chemicals do not circulate; nevertheless, when there is inadequate bloodstream reaching the heart, indicators associated with myocardial injury increase in an expected manner. Within 3 hours of the beginning of chest pain, up to 80% of individuals with a severe MI will have an increase in troponin.

However, not all individuals with cardiac impairment present with obvious symptoms, and thus are unlikely to have had analytic testing. Patients with complicated comorbidities and mild as well as non-specific symptoms, such as unexplained weakness and tiredness, should not be referred to intensive consideration for active recovery. It is therefore prudent for therapists to be aware of the cardiac biomarkers' existence and potential delays in the diagnosis of myocardial ischemia.

Benefit Vs. Risk Considerations of the Therapeutic Intervention

The main consideration while evaluating patient laboratory findings is toward deciding on an appropriate plan of care and comparing the anticipated benefit of therapeutic intervention against the potential danger to the patient.

Physical therapists must carefully predict the physiological changes that may occur when a laboratory value is out of range. They should also be aware of the elevated risk level if a value falls into the critical range. While exercising this type of task in the setting, it is critical to understand suitable laboratory values and the resultant potential of adverse events. Physical therapists should evaluate the possible benefits of a rehabilitative plan that extends the patient's activity when balancing risks and benefits. Immediate risks and benefits, as well as long-term outcomes from the episode of treatment, should be assessed. Collaboration with other members of the inter-professional therapy group is usually required to fully investigate the possible effects of exercise-based recovery intervention. It is consistent and sensible with professional standards for physical therapists to contribute to the creation of facility rules and conventions to aid in clinical decision-making about the use of laboratory values in determining the intensity level of therapy interventions.

What Do My Laboratory Results Mean?

Here are a few things you should know about laboratory results.

1. Unit estimates and ranges for "normal" units might differ from laboratory to laboratory (sometimes up to 30 % contrast).
2. Other factors that influence test results include gender, age, dietary preferences, race, species, amount of exercise, menstrual cycles, use of non-prescription medications (cold medications, aspirin, vitamins, and so on), alcohol consumption, prescription drugs, and specimen collection as well as handling.
3. For the best correlations of laboratory findings, testing should be completed by the same one.
4. Always use the standard ranges indicated on the laboratory report for that specific sample.

5. False-negative and false-positive blood tests are possible. Blood cells will break if they are not properly cared for. If the test components are out of date, they may not function properly. If the temperature isn't quite correct, the results may be skewed as well. Furthermore, if there is a new worker in the laboratory who does not do the test properly, would you put your faith in those outcomes? Certain tests may need to be repeated if you are unsure.
6. Blood test interpretation needs an understanding of the underlying experience and illness process. If your test results are out of the ordinary, we urge that you consult with your primary care physician. It is frequently not the most current result, but the change from a previous test that is typically beneficial in seeking to diagnose a disease.
7. Certain examinations are costlier than others. If you can help the expert understand why a certain test is important for you and they can explain it in their mind, they may justify it to your insurance company and you may obtain your diagnosis sooner, saving money, time, and frustration.
8. There are "rule-outs" for all maladies/diseases. A high or low level in a blood test might be caused by a variety of factors, and they should be "ruled out" by additional observations or tests, as well as hunch and gut intuition. Because of your living habits, age, surroundings, and background, some of the probable consequences will carry greater weight and be more fundamentally suspicious.

Other tests may be used to determine whether a certain disease is "in" or "out" based on the findings of these additional tests for those illnesses that are most likely to be diagnosed. This is similar to completing a jigsaw puzzle and seeking the precise arrangement of its components. Certain clues (puzzle pieces) may fit in one component of the puzzle or another based only on the color of the piece (or your indications for this situation.) You just need to keep trying to see if the piece fits.

Chronic Vs. Acute Considerations of the Therapeutic Intervention

Clinical decisions need an understanding of the patient's symptoms as well as the dynamic physiological changes indicated by the laboratory tests, in addition to comparing a patient's specific laboratory data with established reference ranges for a population. For example, acute laboratory value changes, such as those caused by blood loss from surgery or trauma, may require the physical therapist to implement a more preservationist plan of therapy. Simultaneously, such acute alterations may suggest the possibility of increasingly genuine occurrences contributing to the limited amount of time to physically compensate for this acute change. Patients with prolonged illnesses typically exhibit progressively chronic alterations in laboratory results, which are generally linked to these diseases such as; Congestive Cardiovascular Failure (CHF), Chronic Obstructive Pulmonary Disease (COPD), anemia, or longer-term pharmacological intercessions (e.g., chemotherapy, radiation treatment). Under these circumstances, it is prudent for physical therapists to give the patient time for their body to acclimatize to changes in laboratory values. As a result, this interval time may allow patients to devote more resources to controlling possible adverse events caused by increased cardiorespiratory demand, exercise, and mobility.

Chapter 2: Correct Methods to Obtain Laboratory Samples

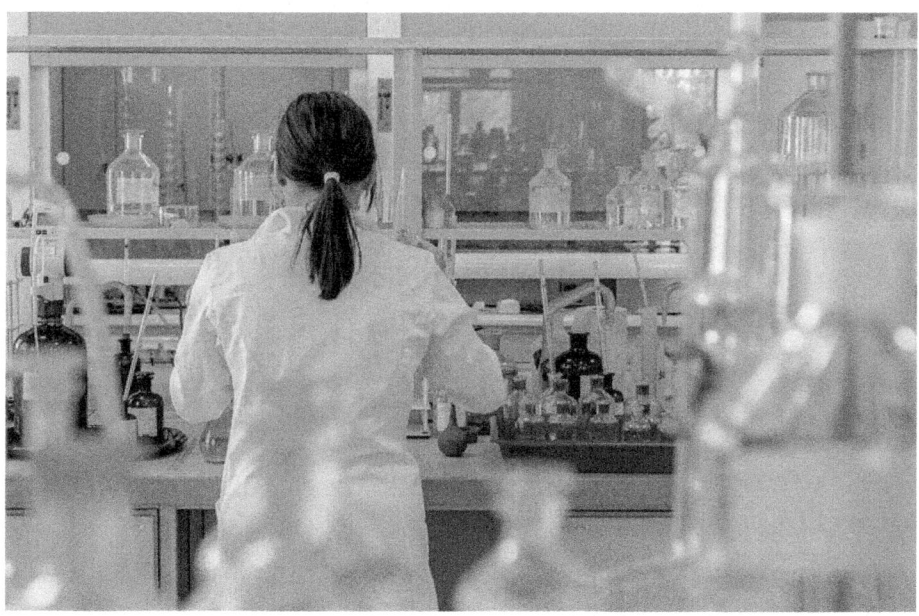

The collecting and management of specimens is an essential element of getting a correct and fast laboratory test result. Specimens must be collected in the appropriate tubes or containers, labeled appropriately, and transferred to the laboratory as soon as possible.

Obtaining Dependable and Precise Laboratory Test Results

Physicians and others are responsible for collecting specimens and delivering them to the laboratory, playing a critical role in ensuring the validity of laboratory test results.

The following are critical precautions for your patients:

1. Avoid mistakes in patient identification

- When providing medicines, blood, or blood components, use at least 2 patient IDs.
- In the presence of the patient, label containers used for blood and other materials.
- Before taking a sample, identify the patient.
- Examine the armbands.
- The patient's complete name, date of birth, or medical record number are all acceptable IDs.

2. Draw the tubes in the correct order

When many tubes are to be taken from a single venipuncture utilizing an evacuated tube system (e.g., BD Vacutainer® or Greiner Vacuette®), there is a proper protocol for blood collection that eliminates cross-contamination of tube additives that might result in incorrect test results. Both plastic and glass blood collection tubes should be labeled as follows.

The following is the order of the draws:

- Blood analysis.

- Tube for coagulation (blue top).
- Serum tube with or without clot activator, gel (red or gold top).
- Heparin tube, either with or without a gel plasma separator (green top).
- EDTA is an abbreviation for Ethyl (purple top, pink top).
- Fluoride and oxalate (gray top).
- Other unique tubes.

All blue tops obtained for coagulation tests that do not include a blood culture must be preceded by the collection of a discard tube. This should be another blue top tube that holds more than 1 ml of blood.

Immediately after collection, all tubes must be gently inverted 10 times end-to-end.

3. Use proper collecting containers

Certain analyses require the use of containers having preservatives and/or anticoagulants, whereas others do not. Using the incorrect container frequently results in incorrect outcomes. Exact requirements may be found in the test catalog.

4. Immediately after collection, gently invert all tubes 10 times

5. Do not transfer specimens from one type of container to another

Specimens must be presented to the laboratory in the same container used for collection.

6. Submit specimens to the laboratory as soon as possible

The analytes separation from blood cells is required for accurate analytes detection in serum or plasma. Analytes move between cells and plasma or serum when they are not separated, as well as glucose is eaten. At room temperature, several analytes are unstable. Drawing additional tubes of blood on patients and keeping them on hand as a backup in case of an unexpected need for more testing might result in incorrect findings and is a risky practice that should be avoided.

For Specimens Collected Away from Campus

To allow full clotting, red and gold top tubes must be left in for 30 minutes. They must then be centrifuged, sorted, and refrigerated until they arrive at the laboratory. Check the instructions for particular test information to see if serum should be frozen.

Purple top CBC tubes can be stored at room temperature for up to 8 hours. Refrigerate for 8 hours till delivery. Greater than 8 hours refrigerate up to 24 hours. Please check particular test stability for tests drawn in purple top tubes other than CBCs.

The handling of green top tubes is determined on the individual test requested. Examine the exact test instructions.

Laboratory Specimen Storage Temperature Requirements

Storage Method	Centigrade (Celsius) Temperature Range
Refrigerated	2 to 8 °C
Frozen	less than or equal to 20 °C
Room/ Ambient	20 to 25 °C

1. Avoid hemolysis

Certain analytes (LD, AST, K, ALT) are found in much greater concentrations in erythrocytes than in plasma. When red cells are hemolyzed, these analytes are released and plasma is diluted, resulting in incorrect laboratory results. Hemolysis may also interfere with analytical methods.

2. *Drawing samples from a line*

If the sample is to be obtained from a line, draw roughly 5 to 10 ml with a first "flush" syringe for adults (20 ml to clear any heparin from the line if coagulation tests are desired). Then, for the necessary tests, draw the syringe. If necessary, the "flush" may be given back to the patient.

Samples Eliminated from the Body Naturally

Samples like feces, urine, and sputum, can be gathered since the body removes them spontaneously, but the patient can collect semen. Some samples from small children or individuals with physical restrictions may need help. Obtaining these samples is usually painless, but it can be difficult and unpleasant at times since it involves the expulsion of physiological wastes and involves body areas and functions that individuals want to keep private.

These sorts of samples can sometimes be taken at home and delivered to a medical office or facility, but they can also be gathered at a medical facility like a doctor's office, clinic, laboratory patient care center, or hospital. These facilities are often intended to minimize patient sample handling and humiliation. You might discover a "pass-through" window in the bathroom, for example, so you don't have to travel down the hall with a see-through container you've just filled up with liquid. It may be a good idea to have instructions printed out and posted on how to get urine or stool samples in the restroom. This way a nurse doesn't have to awkwardly explain how to obtain a "clean-catch" of pee or a fecal sample. If you are worried about these concerns and wish to select a healthcare practitioner or testing facility that offers such choices, you may inquire about their processes, layout, and efforts taken by the staff to protect patient privacy and comfort.

The sorts of samples commonly obtained by the patient are listed below. All sample collecting procedures must be strictly followed. Before you collect your specimen, make sure you understand the instructions.

Examples

Semen

Male patients ejaculate into a specimen receptacle while avoiding the use of lubricants, condoms, or other potentially contaminated items. Typically, males must abstain from ejaculating for at least 2 days but no more than 7 days before collecting the specimen. It must not be refrigerated but should be kept as close to body temperature as possible by keeping it in a pocket and sending it to the laboratory within 60 minutes.

Sputum

Patients are taught to cough out sputum from as deep as possible in the lungs. (In some cases, a health practitioner may be able to aid the patient.) This is best done first thing in the morning before drinking or eating, by taking some deep breaths and then expectorating into the collecting cup. Sputum should be reasonably thick and not as watery as when saliva is produced.

Stool

Patients generally collect this sample themselves when toileting, following instructions to avoid contamination from other materials in the toilet bowl. Patients may also be instructed to refrain from eating specific foods throughout the testing time. They may be asked to collect the sample in a container, place a little quantity into a vial or you can put a small amount on the specific test paper, depending on the test. After handling the sample, thoroughly wash your hands.

Urine

The patient urinates into a container or receptacle to collect the majority of urine specimens. To prevent contamination of the sample by objects outside the urinary system, patients are instructed to clean the genital region and empty a little amount of urine before collecting the specimen into the container. (If a urinary catheter is necessary, the insertion is typically the responsibility of a health practitioner.) The collection of the urine samples is difficult but not unpleasant in itself (An infection, however, can create a burning sensation during urination.). Certain tests require 24-hour urine samples to be obtained at home and frozen during the collection phase. Remember to wash your hands thoroughly after obtaining the specimen.

Saliva

This sort of sample can be obtained using a swab, or if a greater volume is required for testing, patients can be encouraged to expectorate into a container without producing sputum.

Oral fluid

This is a mixture of saliva and oral mucosal transudate (material passing the buccal mucosa from capillaries) collected from the mouth. A fast HIV test, for example, makes use of oral fluids. The sample is collected by the patient using a specific instrument to swab around their outer gums.

Sweat

This sort of sample can be collected utilizing a painless sweat stimulation method that collects fluids onto a plastic coil of tubing, or a piece of gauze or filter paper. The quantity of chloride in the perspiration is then determined. Elevated chloride levels point to a cystic fibrosis diagnosis.

Simple-to-Obtain Specimens

Some samples are obtained simply by wiping the afflicted region with a swab. This sort of procedure can be done at a clinic, your doctor's office, or at the hospital bedside. The sample might be sent to a laboratory for testing (although a few tests can provide in-office results in just a few minutes). Throat, nasal, vaginal, and superficial wound cultures are collected in this manner, for example. While the treatments can be painful at times, they are typically fast, painless, and have no side effects.

Examples

Female reproductive system secretions and tissues

Vaginal secretions are collected by rubbing a cotton swab over the vaginal walls; cervical cells for a Pap test are collected using a cotton swab and spatula or a small brush. Endometrial tissue samples are collected by inserting a thin, flexible, hollow tube into the uterus, which may cause a minor pinching sensation or short discomfort. During this treatment, patients may experience mental and physical distress. The healthcare provider's attentive approach substantially adds to the patient's emotional comfort. If you are experiencing physical discomfort, speak with your healthcare practitioner.

Fluids and secretions from the nose or throat

The material is obtained by wiping the region of interest using a swab and then processed for testing, such as cultures. People generally react to swabbing their throats with a brief "gag" response. If the throat is irritated, the sample collection, no matter how quick, might be painful. Similarly, a nasal swab may be unpleasant since it is inserted and reaches places within the nose that are rarely touched. Remember that the discomfort is just brief, and ask your practitioner if there are some techniques to reduce any soreness that may occur.

Open wounds and sores samples

If the wound or sore is on the skin's outer layer, the specimen is generally collected on a swab by sweeping it over the area and collecting a fluid sample or pus. Touching the open wound area may be uncomfortable at first since the wound is likely to be tender and irritated. However, if the incision or infection is deep, a needle and syringe may be used to extract a sample from the location.

Other
- Hair (for nicotine/cotinine testing, heavy metals, fungal, and drug testing).
- Clippings of fingernails (e.g., for heavy metals and fungal testing).

Samples from Within

Some samples can only be acquired by piercing the body's protective layers (e.g., skin). Blood samples are collected via minimally invasive techniques performed by professionally trained physicians, nurses, or medical workers. Tissue specimen collection is a more complicated technique that may require the use of a local anesthetic to get a sample.

Due to the nature of these collecting procedures, there may be some pain or discomfort associated. Knowing what the technique entails may help to reduce some of the anxiety associated with having to endure these sorts of sample collections.

Examples

Blood

Trained phlebotomists or medical professionals can take blood samples from blood vessels (capillaries, veins, and occasionally arteries). The sample is collected via needle puncture and suction through it into a specific collecting tube. Some specimens can be collected by a finger puncture that results in a drop of blood, such as that used for glucose testing. The process normally takes only a few minutes and causes only little discomfort, usually when the needle is placed or a lancet is punctured.

Tissue biopsy

Tissue samples can be collected from a variety of bodily locations, including the breast, lung, lymph node, and skin. Some pain or discomfort may occur depending on the place and degree of invasiveness. The needed time to execute the operation and recover might also vary considerably. These operations are carried out by healthcare professionals who have received specific training.

Tissue biopsies can be obtained by techniques such as:

Needle biopsy

A needle is introduced into the location, and cells or fluids are extracted with a syringe. At the point of needle insertion, you may feel a small pinch. Typically, recovery time is not necessary, and only a little soreness may be felt afterward.

An excisional biopsy

It is a small surgical technique that involves making an incision and removing a portion or all of the tissue from the location. A closed biopsy is a technique in which a tiny incision is created and an instrument is introduced to assist the surgeon in guiding the sample to the right spot. Typically, these biopsies are done in a hospital operating room. Depending on the operation, a local or general anesthetic is given to keep the patient comfortable. When general anesthesia is administered, recovery time might range from one to several hours.

Cerebrospinal Fluid (CSF)

A lumbar puncture, often known as a spinal tap, is used to collect a sample of cerebrospinal fluid. It is a unique common technique. It is done when the individual is laying on their side, curled up, in a fetal posture, or occasionally seated. An antiseptic is used to clean the back, and a local anesthetic is injected beneath the skin. Through it, between two vertebrae, and into the spinal canal, a specific needle is introduced. The health practitioner collects a tiny amount of CSF in many sterile vials, withdraws the needle, and applies a sterile bandage and pressure to the puncture site. To avoid a headache after the test, the patient will be urged to rest quietly in a flat posture without raising their head for one or more hours. The lumbar puncture technique typically takes less than 30 minutes. The discomfort degree might vary considerably. When the needle is inserted, the most typical sensation is pressure. Inform your doctor if you have a headache or other unusual symptoms, such as discomfort, numbness, tingling in the legs, or feeling pain at the puncture site.

Additional Bodily Fluids

Other bodily fluids, such as synovial, peritoneal, pleural, and pericardial fluids, are collected in the same way as CSF is, by aspirating a sample of the fluid through a needle into a collecting vessel. These are often more complicated collections that need considerable patient preparation, the administration of a local anesthetic, and a period of rest following sample collection.

Bone marrow

A skilled healthcare professional performs the bone marrow aspiration and/or biopsy procedure. Both sorts of samples are often obtained from the hip bone (iliac crest). In rare cases, it can be extracted from the breastbone (sternum). Before the operation, almost all patients are given a light sedative and then instructed to lay on their stomach or side for the act of collection. The location is cleansed with an antiseptic and a local anesthetic is administered as if it were a regular surgical area. The health practitioner puts a needle through the skin and into the bone once the location has become numb. A syringe is connected to the needle during an aspiration, and bone marrow fluid is aspirated. A specific needle is used to capture a core (a cylindrical sample) of bone and marrow for a biopsy.

Even though the patient's skin has been made numb, he or she may experience short but unpleasant pressure (such as pulling or pushing) sensations in the midst of these operations. After the needle is taken out, a sterile bandage is put to the wound, and pressure is administered. The operation may be performed on the other hip (bilateral bone marrow) in some cases, most commonly as part of the initial diagnostic workup. The patient is then told to rest quietly for 48 hours until their blood pressure, heart rate, and temperature return to normal, as well as keeping the collection site dry and covered.

Amniotic Fluid

Amniocentesis is a process that collects a sample of amniotic fluid to discover and diagnose specific birth defects, genetic disorders, as well as chromosomal abnormalities in a fetus. During pregnancy, amniotic fluid surrounds, protects, and nourishes the developing fetus. A sample of amniotic fluid (approximately 1 ounce) is aspirated by introducing a tiny needle through the stomach and uterus into the amniotic sac, this serves to collect both cellular and chemical components that are examined to detect any genetic abnormalities.

Chapter 3: Hematological Tests

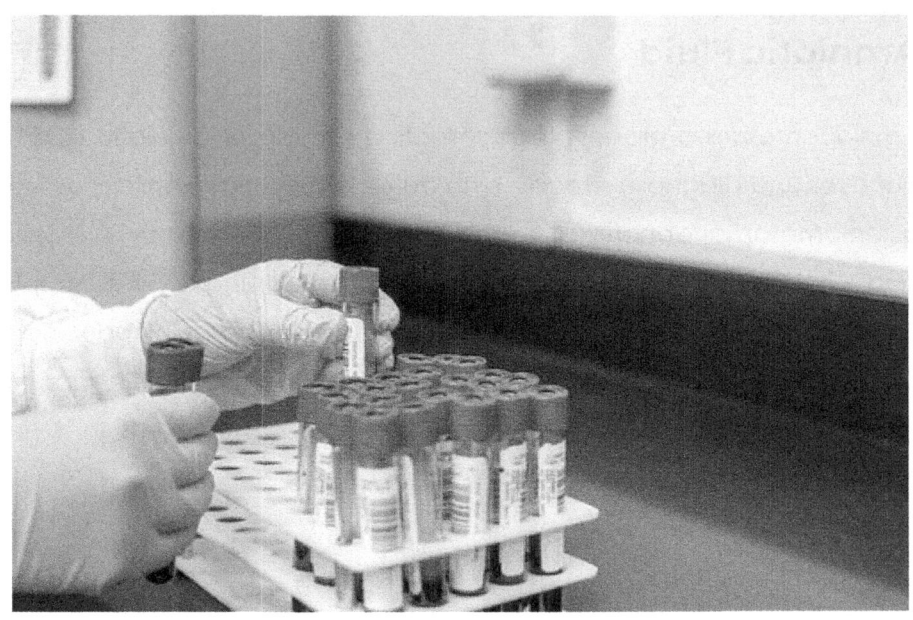

Hematology is the study of blood and its related problems. Hematologists and hematopathologists are highly trained healthcare providers that specialize in blood and blood component disorders. Its cells and bone marrow are included. Hematological testing can assist in the diagnosis of hemophilia, anemia, infection, leukemia, and blood clotting problems.

Hematology is the study of blood, especially how blood might impact overall well-being or illness. Hematology tests recall blood, blood proteins, and blood-creating organs testing.

These tests can evaluate a variety of blood disorders such as anemia, inflammation, infection, blood-clotting problem, leukemia, hemophilia, and the body's response to chemotherapy treatments. Tests may be performed regularly, or they may be relied upon to diagnose actual problems in emergencies. In general, the results of a blood test can provide a detailed assessment of bodily conditions and how inner or exterior conditions may influence a patient's well-being.

This chapter will explain some of the most common hematological tests and what they are used for.

Test: Total Hemoglobin (Hgb or Hb)

A test that measures the quantity of hemoglobin in the blood. Hgb is the pigment component of the erythrocyte and the oxygen-carrying component of blood.

Normal Values:
Males: 12 to17 g/100 ml
Females: 11 to 15 g/100 ml

Clinical implications

Anemia is indicated by a low hemoglobin level. When calculating total blood Hgb, estimates of Hgb in each RBC are somewhat relevant. However, hemoglobin levels are considerably more affected by the overall number of RBCs. In other words, the quantity of RBCs is just as essential as the hemoglobin level in diagnosing anemia.

The amount of hemoglobin in the blood has become a "routine" laboratory test for the majority of patients admitted to hospitals nowadays. Hgb levels are significant in the diagnosis of anemia and bleeding. It is also useful in the diagnosis of several lesser-known illnesses.

Fetal Hemoglobin

Fetal Hb (Hb F) is a common Hb product seen in a fetus's red blood cells and has lesser levels in newborns. It accounts for 50 to 90 % of hemoglobin in newborns; the Hb remainder in adults is made up of HbA1 and HbA2.

Under normal circumstances, the body stops producing fetal Hb around the first year of life and begins producing adult Hb. If this transition does not occur and fetal Hb continues to compose more than 5% of the hemoglobin after 6 months, a problem, notably thalassemia, should be investigated.

Hemoglobin Type and Distribution Variations (in Adults)

Percentage of total Hemoglobin	Hemoglobin	Clinical Implications
Hb A	95% to 100%	Normal
Hb A2	4% to 5.8%	b-thalassemia minor
	1.5% to 3%	b-thalassemia major
	Under 1.5%	b-d-thalassemia minor
Hb F	Under 2%	Normal
	2% to 5%	b-thalassemia minor
	10% to 90%	b-thalassemia major
	5% to 15%	b-d-thalassemia minor
	5% to 35%	Heterozygous hereditary Persistence of fetal Hb (HPFH)
	100%	Homozygous HPFH
	15%	Homozygous Hb S
Homozygous Hb S	70% to 98%	Sickle Cell disease
Homozygous Hb C	90% to 98%	Hb C disease
Heterozygous Hb C	24% to 44%	Hb C trait

Test: Hemoglobin Electrophoresis

Hemoglobin electrophoresis is the most helpful laboratory procedure for separating and quantifying normal and certain aberrant hemoglobin. Different kinds of hemoglobin are separated by electrophoresis to create a succession of bands of color in a medium (which is cellulose acetate or a starch gel). The results are then compared to those of a control sample.

Hb A (also known as Hb A1), Hb A2, Hb S, Hb C, and Hb F are commonly tested, although the laboratory may modify the medium or its pH to broaden the test's range. This test detects normal and abnormal hemoglobin forms, aids in the diagnosis of thalassemia, and helps in the identification of sickle cell disease or trait by evaluating the different types of hemoglobin.

** See the chart above for typical reference values.

Test: Hematocrit (Hct)

The hematocrit is a percentage of packed red blood cells in a whole blood sample measured by volume. An HCT of 40%, for example, implies that a 100 ml sample of blood contains 40 ml of blood cells. Packing is accomplished by centrifuging anti-coagulated whole blood in a capillary tube until the cells are firmly packed and hemolysis is avoided.

Normal Healthy Values:
Males: 40 to 50%
Females: 37 to 47%

Clinical implications

Both small blood samples are collected and compared. They contain the same amount of blood. After then, one specimen is centrifuged and compared to the first. This comparison is then converted into a percentage. The hematocrit, Hct, is used in this comparison. Its value is proportional to the number of RBCs. If the Hct is abnormal, the RBC count may also be irregular. If it is normal, the average size of the RBC is most likely too tiny. The Hct can be reduced by shock, bleeding, dehydration, or excessive IV fluid delivery.

Test: Red Blood Cell Count (RBC count)

A count of the actual (or projected) number of RBCs in one cubic millimeter of whole blood.

Normal Healthy Values:
Males: 4.5 to 6.0 million/cu mm
Females: 4.0 to 5.5 million/cu mm

Clinical implications

The RBC count can be used to diagnose issues including anemia and bleeding. It can be extremely beneficial for diagnosis when combined with other hematological tests. This test can also provide an estimate of hemoglobin levels in the blood. RBCs are short for "Red Blood Corpuscles" (non-nucleated cells). The term corpuscle refers to a mature Red Blood Cell. Only when the immature cell has developed it is capable of transporting oxygen. It is no longer "technically" a cell at that point. When a cell matures, it loses its nucleus and is no longer considered a cell. It would be referred to as a corpuscle. However, they are still referred to as RBCs by everyone (cells). The samples were obtained from whole blood, capillary, or venous blood.

Test: Red Cell Indices (Wintrobe Indices)

A report on the RBC's features listed below is used to diagnose anemia. Anemias can be classified as macrocytic, microcytic, hypochromic, or others if aberrant findings are present. When this is identified, the specific cause of the anemia can be more easily determined.

The following are all indexes:

1. MCV
2. MCH
3. MCHC

1. MCV — Mean corpuscular volume

It is the volume of the average Red Blood Cell.

You calculate it by:

$$\frac{Hct \times 10}{\# \text{ of RBCs}} = MCV$$

Normal Healthy Values: 80 to 94 u3 (cubic microns)

Clinical implications

The MCV represents the relative size of the RBCs. It indicates nothing more about the cell. There are 2 forms of anemia: microcytic and macrocytic anemias. This test can point the doctor in the direction of anemias that affect MCV findings.

   a. Microcytic anemia is a decreased amount of MCV (small cells)

   b. Macrocytic anemia is an increased amount of MCV (large cells)

2. MCH — *Mean corpuscular hemoglobin*

(The weight of the hemoglobin within each cell).

You can calculate it by the following:

$$\frac{Hgb \times 10}{\# \text{ of RBCs}} = MCH$$

Normal Healthy Values: 27 to 31 uug (micro micro-g)

3. MCHC — *Mean corpuscular hemoglobin concentration*

It refers to the amount of hemoglobin in the average RBC.

You can calculate it by the following:

$$\frac{Hgb \times 10}{Hct} = MCHC$$

Clinical implications

The MCHC is affected by RBC size as well as the quantity of hemoglobin in each cell. Certain illnesses and anemias make changes in RBC count and/or hemoglobin content in the cell. The MCHC is less affected by the RBC count than the other tests in this area. As a result, the MCHC can be beneficial in diagnosing diseases that are not dependent on the number of RBCs.

Test: Reticulocyte Count (Retic count)

This is a test that estimates the number of reticulocytes in the blood. The immature RBCs are known as reticulocytes.

Normal Healthy Values: approximately 1% of a normal RBC count (50.000); Results can vary within a range from 0.5 to 1.5%

Clinical implications

Reticulocyte count is a measure of the bone marrow's ability to produce RBCs. A rise over normal generally implies that the body is reacting to pathologies such as hemorrhage, anemia, hemolysis, or another illness process. A low Reticulocyte count might be a sign of aplastic anemia or another illness.

Test: Sickle Cell Test

The Hb S test, commonly known as the sickle cell test, is used to identify sickle cells, which are severely distorted, stiff erythrocytes that can impede blood flow. Sickle cell trait (defined by heterozygous Hb S) is nearly entirely prevalent in African descent persons. It is found in roughly 8% of African Americans.

Test: Iron and Total Iron-Binding Capacity

Iron is required for the production and hemoglobin's function, as well as a variety of other heme and non-heme molecules. Iron is transferred to several bodily compartments for production, storage, and transport once it is absorbed by the gut. Serum iron content is typically greatest in the morning and gradually decreases during the day. As a result, the sample should be taken in the morning.

The amount of iron transferred into someone's blood plasma is measured using an iron assay. Total iron-binding capacity (TIBC) is the iron quantity that would be present in plasma if all transfer was iron-saturated.

Normal Healthy Values:

Serum Iron:
Males: 50 to 50 u/g/dL
Females: 35 to 145 ug/dL

TIBC, or Total Iron-binding capacity:
Both sexes: 250 to 400 ug/dL

Saturation:
Both sexes: 14% to 50%

Test: Ferritin

Ferritin is a protein that stores iron in reticuloendothelial cells. It is typically found in trace amounts in serum. Serum ferritin levels in healthy people are directly proportional to the quantity of accessible iron stored in the body and may be reliably determined using radioimmunoassay.

Normal Healthy Values:

Men: 20 to 300 NG/ml

Women: 20 to 120 NG/ml

6 months to 15 years	7 to 140 NG/ml
2 to 5 months	50 to 200 NG/ml
1 month old	200 to 600 NG/ml
Neonates	25 to 200 NG/ml

The normal serum ferritin level varies with age. Remember to verify with your laboratory because normal levels may change between laboratories. The blood is drawn through venipuncture and placed in a standard 10 ml red-top tube. A blood sample at random is utilized. Except for describing the operation, no additional instructions should be given to the patient. Recent blood transfusions may cause serum ferritin levels to rise.

These levels that are higher than normal may suggest acute or chronic hepatic illness, iron overload, leukemia, Hodgkin's disease, chronic hemolytic anemia, and acute or chronic infection and inflammation, Ferritin levels that are slightly elevated or normal may suggest chronic renal illness.

Serum ferritin levels that are low may suggest chronic iron shortage.

Test: ESR — Erythrocyte Sedimentation Rate

The ESR determines how long it takes for erythrocytes from a whole blood sample to settle the bottom of a vertical tube. The volume of red cells, the surface area, density, aggregation, and the surface charge are all factors that influence the ESR. The sample must be inspected within 2 hours after collection and handled gently; no clotting of the sample is permitted.

Normal Healthy Values: 0 to 20 mm/hr (this will gradually increase along with age).

The ESR is a sensitive yet non-specific test commonly used to detect illness early on. It frequently increases considerably in chronic inflammatory diseases caused by infection or autoimmune origins. Such increases can last for a long time in cases of localized inflammation and cancer.

Increased ESR: may be caused by pregnancy, acute or chronic inflammation, TB, rheumatic fever, paraproteinemia, rheumatoid arthritis, certain cancers, or anemia.

Reduced ESR: This might be due to polycythemia, sickle cell anemia, hyperviscosity, or a low plasma protein level.

Test: Osmotic Fragility

The resistance of red blood cells (RBCs) to hemolysis when exposed to a series of increasingly dilute saline solutions is measured by osmotic fragility. The faster hemolysis begins, the more osmotic fragility the cells have.

This test is used to examine for thalassemia and hereditary spherocytosis (HS). Red blood cells in thalassemia and hereditary spherocytosis are more fragile than usual.

Normal results: The tonicity of the saltwater determines the osmotic fragility values (% of RBCs hemolyzed).

The following are the reference values for the various tonicities:

0.5 g/dL of a sodium chloride (NaCl) solution (un-incubated)
Males: 0.5% to 24.7% hemolysis
Females: 0% to 23.1% hemolysis

0.6 g/dL sodium chloride solution (incubated)
Males: 18% to 55.2% hemolysis
Females: 2.2% to 59.3% hemolysis

0.65 g/dL sodium chloride solution (incubated)
Males: 4% to 24.8% hemolysis
Females: 0.5% to 28.9% hemolysis

0.75 g/dL sodium chloride solution (incubated)
Males: 0.5% to 8.5% hemolysis
Females: 0.1% to 9.3% hemolysis

Low osmotic fragility (this is increased resistance to hemolysis) is a feature of thalassemia, iron deficiency anemia, and other red blood cell diseases characterized by the presence of codocytes (target cells) and leptocytes. It can also develop with splenectomy.

High osmotic fragility (increased propensity to hemolysis) occurs in genetic spherocytosis, autoimmune hemolytic anemia, severe burns, chemical poisoning, or neonatal hemolytic illness (erythroblastosis fetalis).

Test: WBC Count — White Blood Cell Count (Leukocyte Count)

This is a laboratory test that records the number of white blood cells (WBCs).

Normal Healthy Values: total WBC: 4.500 to 10.500

Basic Types of WBC

- Neutrophils (Granulocyte)
- Lymphocytes (Non-Granulocyte)
- Monocytes (Non-Granulocyte)
- Eosinophils (Granulocyte)
- Basophils (Granulocyte)

Clinical implications

White Blood Cells, as we all know, are our bodies' first line of defense against invading germs and the majority of other dangerous organisms. This test (WBC) counts the total number of WBCs of all kinds. A closer look at the varied types and quantities of cells present might reveal a lot about the condition of the body's defensive system. On any one day, the White Blood Cells count might fluctuate by up to 2.000.

Test: Differential Cell Count Also Known as "Diff" or "Differential"

A laboratory test that counts actual numbers of WBC's different types.

Clinical implications

The chart below shows the normal levels for each kind of WBC. The overall number of WBCs must always be considered when interpreting differential data.

The white blood cell differential assesses the distribution and shape of them. As a result, it gives more detailed information about a patient's immune system than a WBC count alone. The differential test involves the laboratory classifying 100 or more white cells on a stained film of peripheral blood into 2 primary kinds of leukocytes.

They are as follows:

1. Granulocytes (neutrophils, eosinophils, basophils).
2. Non-Granulocytes (lymphocytes, monocytes).

The proportion of each kind is then calculated.

WBC Levels

CELL TYPE	ADULT VALUE	ABSOLUTE VALUE	RELATIVE VALUE (6 to 18 years old)	
			BOYS	GIRLS
Neutrophils	47.6% to 76.8%	1,950 to 8,400/ul	38.5% to 71.5%	41.9% to 76.5%
Lymphocytes	16.2% to 43%	660 to 4,600/ul	19.4% to 51.4%	16.3% to 46.7%
Monocytes	0.6% to 9.6%	24 to 960/ul	1.1% to 11.6%	0.9% to 9.9%
Eosinophils	0.3% to 7%	12 to 760/ul	1% to 8.1%	0.8% to 8.3%
Basophils	0.3% to 2%	12 to 200/ul	0.25% to 1.3%	0.3% to 1.4%

Chapter 4: Serum Electrolytes Tests

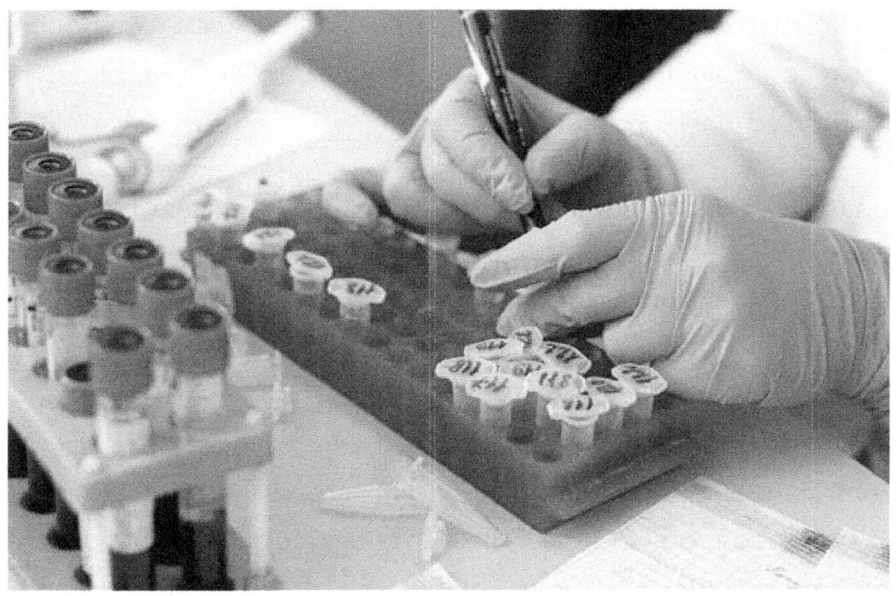

Electrolytes are minerals required for the most basic bodily functions. Serum electrolytes are used to assess individuals who have electrolyte and acid-base abnormalities. Serum electrolyte panels are routinely ordered and contain serum potassium, sodium, chloride, and serum bicarbonate.

Electrolytes are ionized elements in a solution that moves in an electric field. Depending on whether they move toward the cathode or the anode, they are referred to as either cations or anions. Sodium, potassium, calcium, and magnesium are the most common cations present in bodily fluids. Chloride, bicarbonate, phosphate, and sulfate are the most common anions present in bodily fluids.

Other compounds in the bodily fluid that are ionized and carry an electric charge in a solution include certain organic acid radicals like lactate, amino acids, proteins, and many other trace components. Sodium, potassium, chloride, calcium, magnesium, and phosphorus are all discussed in this chapter.

Electrolytes have a role in all bodily functions. They help to maintain appropriate osmotic pressure and water distribution throughout the body, both within cells and in extracellular fluid. They play an important role in numerous metabolic processes. Any electrolyte imbalance will have far-reaching consequences on the body.

Serum potassium is an electrolyte and mineral found in the blood that may be measured via tests. Potassium has a restricted normal range and is essential for cardiac muscle as well as nerve cell function. It is consumed through food and beverages and eliminated mostly through urine. A little amount is excreted via the gastrointestinal system. Potassium deficiency is well-known for producing abnormal heartbeats, often known as arrhythmias.

Serum sodium is frequently tested to determine acid-base and water balance, electrolyte abnormalities, as well as kidney function. Sodium accounts for approximately 95% of the osmotically active chemicals in the extracellular compartment fluid. Sodium is controlled by hormonal factors, and any excess is eliminated by the kidneys, which carefully control extracellular sodium.

Serum chloride is the most abundant anion in the extracellular space. Chloride and its effects on water balance besides osmotic pressure, as well as acid-base balance, help to preserve cellular integrity. Chloride also has a major role in cardiovascular pathophysiology and neuronal pharmacology.

One of the most plentiful components in the adult body is calcium, which accounts for roughly 2% of adult body weight or more than 1 kg. Except for 1%, all calcium in the bones is in the form of calcium hydroxyapatite. The plasma contains all calcium in the blood. About 40% of serum calcium is bound to proteins.

About 10% of the calcium in circulation occurs as inorganic and organic anions of bicarbonate, lactate, and citrate; the remaining 50% is free, known as ionized calcium. Calcium ions are required for the neurological system to operate properly; they also maintain the contractility of the heart and skeletal muscles. Calcium is also linked to blood coagulation and bone mineralization. The calcium content in the blood is carefully regulated by the parathyroid hormone (PTH) and 1.25 hydroxyvitamin D.

Elemental phosphorus is not originated in the body in free form and is only found as a component of organic and inorganic substances. Phosphates, like calcium, are found predominantly in an inorganic form (hydroxyapatite) in human skeletons. Organic chemicals account for around 15% of the total in our soft tissue and circulation.

Laboratory tests determine the amount of biologically bound phosphorus. Magnesium is the most important intracellular cation in the body. Magnesium, along with extracellular calcium, plays an important role in proper neuromuscular function. Furthermore, intracellular magnesium serves as a cofactor for nucleic acids, different enzymes, and transporters required for replication, energy metabolism, and proper cellular function.

Test: Sodium, (Na Serum)

This is a laboratory test that determines the amount of sodium in the blood. This is the most abundant cation in extracellular fluid, and it is known for its ability to hold water.

Normal Values:
Adult: 135 to 145 mEq/L (same for child)
Infants: 134 to 150 mEq/L

Clinical implications

There is no need for any specific patient preparation. However, if the patient has consumed a high-sodium meal in the previous 24 hours, this should be recorded because it may influence the test. A serum sodium test is rarely ordered on its own. This is often ordered as part of a panel of electrolyte testing. The same may be said for the other electrolytes discussed in this section.

This electrolyte performs a variety of tasks in the body, including the conduction of neuromuscular impulses via the sodium pump (sodium moves into cells as potassium moves out for cellular activity), enzyme activity, intravascular fluid osmolality, acid-base balance control, and others.

Decreased levels (hyponatremia) can be induced by a variety of factors, including vomiting, diarrhea, gastric suction, excessive sweating, continuous IV 5 % Dextrose/water; low-sodium diet, burns, inflammatory responses, tissue damage, and others.

Dehydration, severe vomiting and diarrhea, CHF, Cushing's illness, hepatic failure, a high-sodium diet, and other symptoms can be caused by an increase in salt.

Test: Potassium, (K+)

Definition: Serum electrolyte

Normal Values: 3.5 to 5.0 mEq/L

Clinical implications

Potassium is another vital electrolyte in the body. Our bodies are extremely sensitive to aberrant potassium levels. With high or low amounts of this electrolyte, cardiac arrhythmias and neurological problems might occur. Hypokalemia can be induced by a reduction in intake, prolonged vomiting, renal failure, cirrhosis, and other factors. Renal failure, among other things, can induce hyperkalemia. The nurse must closely monitor the vital signs of any patients in the aforementioned risk groups, particularly the cardiac and mental conditions.

Test: Chloride, (Cl)

Definition: Serum electrolyte

Normal Values: 95 to 105 mEq/L

Clinical implications

The chloride anion is mostly present in extracellular fluid. Chloride, like sodium, plays a vital function in fluid balance. Chloride is also crucial in maintaining acid-base equilibrium. However, the chloride test is frequently overlooked; in most situations, if the sodium result is normal, the chloride value will be normal as well. As a result, chloride testing is not done very frequently in certain hospitals. The majority of the chloride consumed is coupled with sodium (sodium chloride-table salt). The average daily chloride consumption is around 2 g.

Test: Serum Osmolality

The total amount of active electrolyte particles in the blood.

Normal Values: Adult: 280 to 300 Osm/kg/H2O.

Clinical implications

The number of dissolved particles in serum is measured by serum osmolality (electrolytes, urea, and sugar). It can aid in the diagnosis of fluid and electrolyte abnormalities. Because of its abundance in the body, sodium contributes approximately 90% of serum osmolality.

There are typically no limitations when it comes to collecting blood. For testing, a random sample is obtained. The serum osmolality will rise as a result of hyperglycemia. Reduced osmolality is linked to serum dilution as a result of over-hydration and excessive fluid intake. A fluid volume deficit, hypovolemia, dehydration, salt overload, or hyperglycemia are all related to increased osmolality. Thirst, dry mucous membranes, low skin turgor, and shock-like symptoms are all associated with high osmolality.

Test: Acid Phosphatase

The test is used to detect prostate cancer and to monitor response to therapy for prostate cancer.

Normal Value:
0 to 1.1 Bodanzky units/ml
1 to 4 King-Armstrong units/ml
0.13 to 0.63 BLB units/ml

Clinical implications

Acid phosphatase is a phosphatase enzyme found predominantly in the prostate gland and sperm. It is also present in other organs, but at minute levels. The 2 primary isoenzymes are prostatic and erythrocytic enzymes. In the laboratory, they may be separated. The prostatic isoenzyme is mainly focused on prostate cancer. The more extensive the tumor, the higher the likelihood of elevated blood acid phosphatase levels.

- **Acid phosphatase levels have significantly increased:** A tumor that has grown outside of the prostatic capsule.
- **Acid phosphatase levels that are somewhat elevated:** Prostatic infarction, Paget's disease, Gaucher's disease, and multiple myeloma are all conditions that affect the prostate.
- **High acid phosphatase levels are decreasing:** Prostatic cancer successfully treated

Fluorides and phosphates have the potential to provide false-negative findings. Clofibrate has the potential to provide false-positive findings. Within 48 hours after the test, prostate massage, catheterization, or rectal examination may interfere with the findings. Hemolysis caused by harsh handling of the sample or poor storage may skew test findings. Acid phosphatase levels decline by 50% in one hour if the sample is left at room temperature without a preservative or is not packed in ice.

Test: Ammonia Measures Plasma Levels of Ammonia

Normal Value: is less than 50 mcg/dL

Clinical implications

This test examines plasma ammonia levels, a non-protein nitrogen molecule that aids in acid-base balance. The majority of ammonia is absorbed from the gastrointestinal system, where it is generated by bacterial activity on protein. The kidneys generate a lower amount of ammonia. The nitrogen portion of ammonia is normally used by the body to generate amino acids. The liver subsequently converts ammonia to urea, which the kidneys excrete.

However, in conditions like cirrhosis of the liver, it can bypass the liver and collect in the circulation. As a result, plasma ammonia levels may aid in determining the degree of hepatocellular injury.

Precautions:

1. Acetazolamide, thiazides, ammonium salts, furosemide, hyperalimentation, and portacaval shunt may all induce a rise in ammonia levels.
2. These may reduce ammonia levels: kanamycin, neomycin, and lactulose.
3. The ammonia test findings may be influenced by hemolysis of the blood sample produced by harsh handling.
4. Make sure the bleeding has stopped before releasing pressure from the venipuncture site. Hepatic illness might cause bleeding to last longer.
5. This test typically requires a fasting specimen; however, random samples may also be utilized (indicate if they are fasting or random).

Increased plasma ammonia levels:

This is seen with individuals who are in a hepatic coma, have Reye's syndrome, severe congestive heart failure, gastrointestinal hemorrhage, or erythroblastosis failure.

Test: Creatinine

It is a test to determine the amount of creatinine in the blood. Creatinine is a non-protein byproduct of creatine oxidation. It is a byproduct of protein metabolism produced by the liver, kidneys, gut, and pancreas. It is a test for determining renal glomerular filtration and screening for renal impairment.

Normal Value:
Males: 0.8 to 1.2 mg/dL
Females: 0.6 to 0.9 mg/dL

Clinical implications

Because renal impairment is essentially the only source of creatinine increase, this test offers a sensitive assessment of renal damage. Creatinine is comparable to creatine, which occurs in serum in proportion to muscle mass. Creatinine, unlike creatine, is readily eliminated by the kidneys with little or no absorption by the tubules. Creatinine levels are thus proportional to the glomerular filtration rate. Because these levels are generally steady, higher levels usually suggest impaired renal function. Elevated serum creatinine levels are most commonly found in people with a renal disease that has severely destroyed 50% or more of the kidney's nephrons.

The sample is collected in a standard red-top 10 ml or 15 ml tube. It is best to avoid eating and drinking for 8 hours before the venipuncture to collect the samples. Ascorbic acid, barbiturates, and diuretics can all make an increase in the blood's creatinine levels. Even in the context of normal renal function, patients with unusually big muscle masses, such as athletes, may have above-average creatinine levels. These levels are also elevated in those with Gigantism and Acromegaly.

If the test is based on the Jaffe reaction, sulfobromophthalein or phenolsulfonphthalein administered during the preceding 24 hours might raise serum creatinine levels.

Chapter 5: Test for Heart Disease

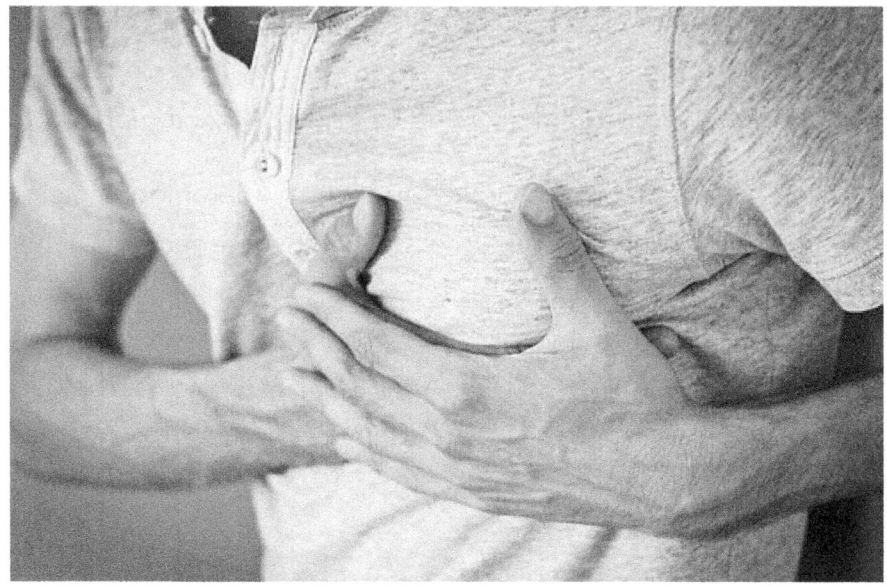

Heart disease refers to any ailment that affects your heart, such as coronary artery infection and arrhythmia. According to the CDC's Trusted Source, heart disease is responsible for one every four deaths in the United States each year. It is the leading cause of death in humans.

Your primary care physician will perform a series of tests and evaluations to identify heart disease. Some of these tests can also be used to check heart disease before you notice any symptoms.

Symptoms of Heart Disease

- Chest pain
- Fainting
- Fast slow heartbeat

- Shortness of breath
- Chest tightness
- Sudden swelling in your feet, abdomen, legs, feet, or ankles

If you experience any of the symptoms listed above, you should schedule an appointment with your primary care physician. Early detection and treatment can significantly reduce your risk of problems such as a stroke or heart attack.

Physical Exam and Blood Tests

During your appointment, your primary care physician will learn about your symptoms and your family's therapy history. They will also take your pulse and blood pressure.

Blood tests may also be ordered by your primary care physician. Cholesterol tests, for example, assess the amount of cholesterol and fat in your bloodstream. These tests can be used by your doctor or specialist to help determine your risk of having a heart attack or developing heart disease.

A total cholesterol test examines 4 types of lipids in your blood:

1. The total cholesterol in your blood is the sum of all the cholesterol in your blood.
2. LDL cholesterol, often known as "bad" cholesterol, is a kind of low-density lipoprotein (LDL) cholesterol. Much of it causes fat to form in your arteries, reducing blood flow. This can result in a heart attack or stroke.
3. High-density lipoprotein (HDL) cholesterol is sometimes referred to as "good" cholesterol. It aids in LDL cholesterol diversion and clearing arteries.

4. Triglycerides are a type of fat found in the blood. Significant triglyceride levels are commonly associated with smoking, diabetes, and excessive alcohol intake.

C-responsive protein (CRP) tests may also be ordered by your primary care physician to evaluate your body for inflammation and symptoms. They can assess your risk of heart disease based on the findings of your CRP and cholesterol testing.

Non-invasive Tests for Heart Disease

Following the completion of a physical examination and blood tests, your doctor may arrange more non-invasive testing. The term "non-invasive" refers to tests that do not use equipment that breaches the skin or physically enters the body. There are several non-invasive tests that your primary care physician can do to detect heart infection.

Electrocardiogram

An electrocardiogram (EKG) is a quick test that detects electrical activity in your heart. This movement is recorded on a paper strip. This test may be used by your primary care physician to look for abnormal heart damage or heartbeat.

Echocardiogram

Echocardiography is a heart ultrasound. It generates a picture of your heart with sound waves. It may be used by your doctor to evaluate your heart muscles and valves.

The stress test

Your primary physician can examine you while you are engaged in vigorous exercise to diagnose cardiac problems. They may ask you to do a few minutes of stationary walking, biking, or running on a treadmill as part of a stress test. As your pulse rate rises, they will assess your body's reaction to stress.

Carotid ultrasound

A carotid duplex scan utilizes pulsed sound waves to photograph the carotid arteries on both sides of your neck. It allows your primary care physician or doctor to monitor the plaque formation in your arteries and assess your risk of stroke.

Holter monitor

If your primary care physician needs to monitor your heart for 24 to 48 hours, they will ask you to wear a Holter monitor. This little gadget functions like a continuous EKG. It can be used by your primary care physician to discover cardiac irregularities that would otherwise go undetected on a standard EKG, such as arrhythmias or erratic heartbeats.

Chest X-ray

A chest X-ray uses a little amount of radiation to create images of your chest, including your heart. This helps your doctor figure out what's causing your chest discomfort or shortness of breath.

Tilt table test

If you've blacked out, your doctor may do a tilt table test. They will suggest that you lie on a table that moves from horizontal to vertical. They'll check your pulse, circulatory strain, and oxygen saturation while the table moves. The results might help your primary care physician determine if you are blacking out was caused by a heart infection or another issue.

A CT scans

A CT scan is a very useful procedure that uses a series of X-ray images to create a cross-sectional image of your heart. To diagnose cardiac problems, your doctor may use a variety of CT scans. They may, for example, use a calcium score screening heart scan to look for calcium deposits in your coronary veins. Alternatively, they may use coronary CT angiography to look for calcium or fat deposits in your arteries.

MRI of the heart

Huge radio and magnet waves create images of your body within an MRI. An expert takes images of your veins and heart while it is pulsing during a cardiac MRI. Following the test, your primary care physician can use the images to detect a variety of problems, including coronary artery disease and heart muscle infections.

Invasive Tests to Diagnose Heart Disease

Noninvasive testing does not always provide sufficient information. To identify a heart infection, your primary care physician may need to use an invasive approach. Instruments that physically penetrate the body, such as a needle, scope, or tube, are used in invasive methods.

Coronary angiography and cardiac catheterization

During cardiac catheterization, a doctor inserts a flexible, long tube into a vein in your groin or another region of your body. At that moment, doctors will insert this tube into your heart. It can be used by your primary care physician to conduct a test looking for cardiac irregularities and blood vessel problems.

Catheterization, for example, may be used to complete a coronary angiography. They'll inject a rare dye into the veins of your heart. After that, they'll use an X-ray to examine your coronary arteries. This test can be used to look for blocked or constricted arteries.

Electrophysiology study

If you have irregular cardiac rhythms, your doctor may order an electrophysiological study to discover the cause and the best treatment strategy for you. During this test, your primary care physician inserts a terminal catheter into a vein in your leg and into your heart. This electrode is used to deliver electric signals to your heart and provide a roadmap for its electrical movement.

Your doctor may suggest medicines or various medications to try to restore your normal heart rhythm.

When to see your doctor

Make an appointment with your doctor if you suspect have a heart infection or illness.

The following factors increase your risk of developing a heart infection:

- History of smoking.
- Poor diet.
- Age.
- Family history of heart disease.
- Obesity.

Your primary care physician may perform a physical examination, order blood tests, or use other procedures to look for problems with your heart or veins. These tests can help them diagnose coronary artery disease and develop a treatment strategy.

Heart failure and stroke are two complications of heart disease. Early detection and treatment can reduce the risk of problems. If you have any concerns, speak with your healthcare provider. They'll teach you how to recognize the symptoms of a heart infection and maintain a healthy heart.

Common Medical Tests to Diagnose Heart Conditions

Your primary care physician may order a variety of medical tests to assist determine the nature of your cardiac issue and the best way to treat it. A part of these tests is explained further down.

Blood tests

When your muscle is injured, such as in heart failure, your body releases chemicals into your blood. They can detect the chemicals and determine whether or not your heart muscle has been damaged, as well as the extent to which it has been destroyed.

Blood tests are also performed to determine the levels of various chemicals in your blood, such as triglycerides and cholesterol), minerals, and vitamins.

A vein in your arm is used to draw blood for the test. A laboratory then tests it and transmits the results to your primary care physician, who will inform you of the findings.

Electrocardiogram (ECG)

An ECG examines the electrical forces that drive your heart. It demonstrates how well your heart is beating.

Small sticky wire and dot leads are attached to your arms, chest, and legs. Leads are connected to an ECG machine, which records and prints the electrical driving forces.

An ECG may be used by your doctor to diagnose heart failure or abnormal heart rhythms (called 'arrhythmias').

Exercise stress test

A stress test, often known as the 'exercise' or 'treadmill' test, is a type of ECG that is performed while you exercise. It can help your doctor figure out how well your heart works when you're physically engaged.

Echocardiogram (ultrasound)

A typical test is an echocardiography. It creates a picture of your heart using ultrasound, which is similar to an X-ray. It employs a test on your chest or down your spine (throat).

It allows your primary care physician to determine if there are any problems with your heart's chambers and valves, as well as how well your heart pumps blood.

Nuclear cardiac stress test

This test is also known as 'a thallium scan, ' or a 'dual-isotope treadmill.'

A radioactive material known as a 'tracer' is injected into your circulatory system. It travels to your heart and releases energy. Excellent cameras capture this energy from outside the body.

Your primary care physician will use this picture to determine how much blood flows to your heart muscle and how well your heart pumps blood while you are resting and moving. This test also allows your doctor to determine whether your heart muscle has been damaged.

Coronary angiogram

A coronary angiography, often known as a 'cardiac catheterization,' may be performed following angina or a heart attack.

In your arm, groin, or wrist, a catheter (a little tube) is inserted into an artery. The catheter is inserted into the artery and advanced until it reaches your heart.

An unusual color is injected into your coronary arteries, followed by an X-ray.

It demonstrates to your primary care physician where and how much of your coronary arteries are clogged or blocked. It also displays how well your heart is pounding. Coronary angiograms assist your doctor in determining the best course of therapy for you.

Magnetic resonance imaging (MRI)

An MRI uses highly powerful radio and magnetic waves to create detailed heart images on a computer. It can capture both static and moving images of your heart. Occasionally, a different hue is used to make parts of the heart and coronary arteries easier to view.

This test reveals to your primary care physician the structure of your heart and how effectively it functions, allowing them to recommend the best therapy for your needs.

Coronary computed tomography angiogram (CCTA)

This is a computed tomography (CT) scan that may be used to assist diagnose coronary artery disease. It is a non-invasive test for those who are experiencing unusual cardiac side effects.

Blood Tests for Heart Disease

Your blood contains various clues regarding the health of your heart. One of these is if you have elevated levels of what is termed "bad" cholesterol in your blood might indicate that you're at a higher risk of developing heart failure. Furthermore, several chemicals in your blood can help your primary care physician determine if you have heart failure or are at risk for having fatty deposits (plaques) in your veins (atherosclerosis).

Remember that a single blood test does not determine your risk of heart disease. Hypertension, smoking, high cholesterol, and diabetes are the most important risk factors for heart disease.

Below are some of the blood tests that doctors and experts use to detect and treat heart disease.

Test: cholesterol

A cholesterol test, also known as a lipid profile or lipid panel, measures the amount of fat in your blood. Estimates might reveal your chances of getting a heart attack or other cardiac ailment.

Typically, the exam includes estimations of:

- The total amount of cholesterol. This is a measurement of the amount of cholesterol in your blood. A substantial amount increases the risk of heart infection/disease.
- Ideally, your total cholesterol should be less than 200 milligrams per deciliter (mg/dL) or 5.2 millimoles per liter (mmol/L).
- LDL cholesterol is a kind of low-density lipoprotein (LDL) cholesterol. In certain situations, this is referred to as "bad" cholesterol. A high level of LDL cholesterol in your blood causes plaque to form in your arteries, reducing blood flow. These plaque deposits can rupture, causing serious heart and vascular problems.

- A person's LDL cholesterol level should be lower than 130 mg/dL (3.4 mmol/L). Under 100 mg/dL (2.6 mmol/L) is ideal, especially if you have diabetes or a history of cardiovascular failure, a heart stent, surgery, or another heart or vascular disease. The recommended LDL level is less than 70 mg/dL (1.8 mmol/L) in people who are at respiratory high-risk failure.
- HDL cholesterol (high-density lipoprotein). This is sometimes referred to as "good" cholesterol since it helps deflect LDL ("bad") cholesterol, keeping arteries open and blood flowing smoothly.
- Your HDL cholesterol level should be greater than 40 mg/dL (1.0 mmol/L) if you are a guy. Ladies should aim for HDL levels more than 50 mg/dL (1.3 mmol/L).
- Triglycerides are a certain type of fat that is found in the blood. High triglyceride levels usually indicate that you consume more calories than you burn. Significant amounts may increase the risk of heart disease.
- A person's triglyceride level should be less than 150 mg/dL (1.7 mmol/L).
- Cholesterol that is not HDL. The differential between absolute cholesterol and HDL cholesterol in non-high-density lipoprotein cholesterol (non-HDL-C). It contains cholesterol for lipoprotein particles involved in vein solidification. The non-HDL-C component may be a better risk indicator than total cholesterol or LDL cholesterol.

High-sensitivity C-reactive protein

C-reactive protein (CRP) is produced by your liver as part of your body's response to injury or sickness, which produces swelling throughout the body (inflammation).

During atherosclerosis, inflammation plays a crucial role. High-affectability CRP (hs-CRP) testing can assist you to determine your heart infection risk before you develop symptoms. Higher levels of hs-CRP are linked to an increased risk of heart failure, stroke, and cardiovascular disease.

Because CRP levels might be momentarily elevated by a variety of conditions, for example, a cold or going for a previous run, the test should be performed again, 2 weeks apart. An hs-CRP level of more than 2.0 milligrams per liter (mg/L) indicates an increased risk of heart disease.

Consolidating your hs-CRP test and heart disease risk with other blood test results risk factors provides your primary care physician with an overall picture of your heart health. Your doctor will determine if you might benefit from having your hs-CRP calculated to better assess your risk of stroke or heart attack.

Statin medications that lower cholesterol may lower CRP levels, lowering your risk of heart disease.

Lipoprotein (a)

Lipoprotein (a), often known as Lp (a), is a kind of LDL cholesterol. Your Lp (a) level is normally determined by your genes and is seldom altered by your lifestyle.

Elevated Lp (a) levels may indicate an increased risk of heart infection, although it is unclear how much risk there is. If you already have heart disease or atherosclerosis but appear to have cholesterol levels in the normal range or if your family has a history of early-onset heart disease, stroke, or sudden death, your primary care physician may schedule an Lp (a) test.

Medications to decrease Lp (a) are being developed; however, it is not yet known what effects reducing Lp (a) will have on the risk of heart infection.

Plasma ceramides

This test determines the levels of ceramides in the blood. They are produced by all cells and play an important role in the growth, function, and eventually death of many tissue types. Lipoproteins transport ceramides through the blood, and they are linked to atherosclerosis.

Three in particular ceramides have been connected to plaque formation in insulin and artery resistance, which can lead to type 2 diabetes. Significant amounts of these ceramides in the blood indicate an increased risk of cardiovascular disease in the next 1 to 5 years.

Natriuretic peptides

Cerebral natriuretic peptide (CNP), also known as B-type natriuretic peptide (BNP), is a protein found in your blood arteries and heart. It allows your body to eliminate fluid, relax veins, and transport sodium into your pee.

When your heart is damaged, the body secretes increased quantities of BNP into the circulatory system in an attempt to alleviate the pressure on your heart. One of the most common applications of BNP is to determine whether shortness of breath is caused by a health problem.

Typical BNP levels vary according to gender, age, and whether or not you are overweight. Setting up a baseline BNP can be beneficial for those who have a health breakdown, and future tests can be used to assess how effectively therapy performs.

N-terminal BNP, a variant of this, is also useful for detecting cardiovascular breakdown and estimating the risk of heart failure and other problems in those who already have heart disease.

A substantial level of BNP alone is insufficient to diagnose a cardiac problem. Your doctor will also evaluate your risk factors and the findings of additional blood tests.

Troponin T

It is a protein present in the heart muscle. Estimating this protein with a high-affectivity troponin T test aids experts in detecting heart failure and determining your risk of coronary illness/heart disease. Increased troponin T levels have been linked to an increased risk of heart disease in those who have no symptoms.

Chapter 6: Serological Tests for Specific Infections

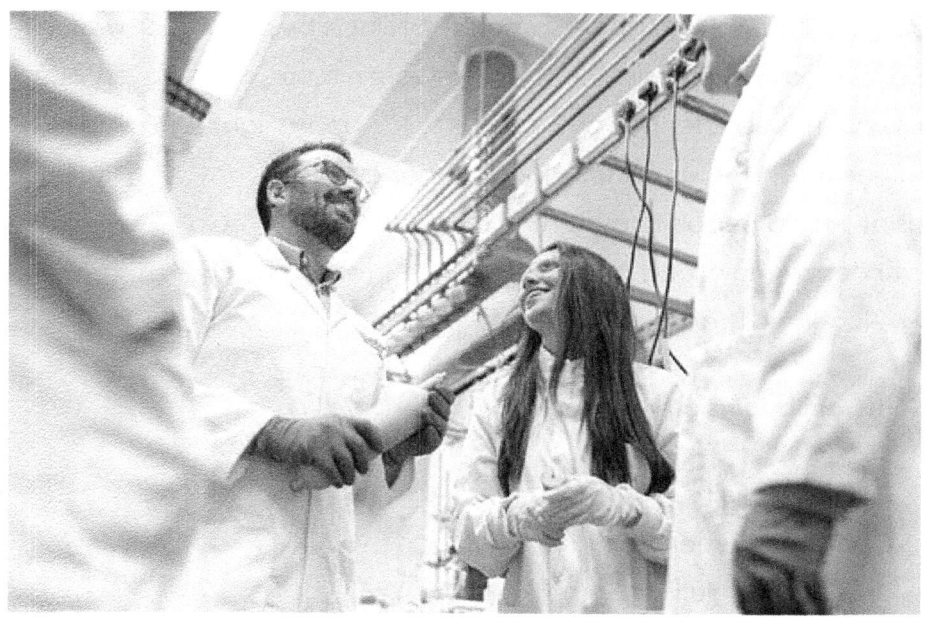

The study of immunological bodies in human blood is known as serology. They are the result of the body's defensive systems against disease-causing pathogens. The antibody-antigen reaction is the central concept in serology. The antigen comes first since it is the substance that "prompts" the body to create antibodies. The antibody, as we all know, is the substance that fights the invading pathogen. Antibodies come in several different forms because antigens can infiltrate into the body in a variety of ways. Serology tests are used to detect whether a person has been exposed to a disease in the past. The tests seek for antibodies produced as part of the immune response that can bind to the virus. COVID-19 serology tests seek for antibodies that bind to particular SARS-CoV-2 proteins (antigens) on the virus.

These proteins are found if a person has been infected and then recovered from the virus. Even after the illness has passed, these tests may be used to estimate the frequency of disease in a community. Serology tests rely on blood samples obtained by a blood draw from a person's arm or a finger stick. These tests are not utilized to identify active COVID-19 because they detect signs of the body's fight against the virus rather than the virus itself. There is not presently any test that can establish if a person is resistant to reinfection by SARS-CoV-2 because it is uncertain how long antibodies will be protective. After all, antibody levels generally decline over time.

Some antibodies are as follows:

- Agglutinins
- Complement-Fixing
- Hemagglutinins
- Opsonins
- Precipitins
- Hemagglutinin Inhibitors
- Cytolysins
- Hemolysins

In this part, we will just cover the most common tests in the field of serology. As we look at these tests and their results, we'll see that many of them rely largely on the fact that the body generates particular antibodies in reaction to specific invading organisms, viruses, proteins, and other foreign elements that assault our bodies.

Serological Examinations

Serological testing is necessary for the identification of various diseases as well as syphilis. Serological tests can be used to diagnose bacterial infections, viral infections, and other illnesses. The following are some of the most prevalent diseases for which serology tests can assist in diagnosis.

Bacterial Infections

Infections caused by dangerous strains of bacteria spread on or within the body, resulting in a bacterial infection. Bacteria have the ability to infect virtually any part of the human body. Among the many ailments that can be brought on by harmful bacteria include pneumonia, meningitis, and food poisoning. In general, bacteria can be categorized as either rod-shaped (bacilli), helical (spirilla), or spherical (cocci). A variety of procedures including genetic analysis are performed to identify bacterial strains and assist doctors decide on the best treatment.

They are the most common type of bacterial infection. Antigens may be easily generated for serological studies using bacterial organism cultures. The agglutination test is the most often utilized test. This test combines the patient's serum, which contains antibodies, with a laboratory-prepared solution of the deadly illness organism.

Because of the antigen-antibody interaction, the mixture will agglutinate, or cluster together. The degree to which they clump not only confirms the original diagnosis, but also indicates the amount of, or concentration of, antibodies present. This test is used to diagnose dysentery, tularemia, and brucellosis of all kinds.

Infections caused by viruses

Certain serology tests can detect the presence of viral infection. It is identical to the bacterial tests mentioned above, but two separate blood samples are required, from two different times in the patient's sickness. When the titer of antibodies rises, a virus can be identified as the source of the illness. As previously stated, the assays utilized include complement-fixation, hemagglutination, and others.

Others

Serological testing can also be used to identify a variety of different diseases. The tests used to diagnose the following diseases are extremely precise. They are unusual diseases, and the findings of these tests, together with other test results, will be used by the M.D. to determine the diagnosis.

1. Atypical primary pneumonia

This disease is diagnosed using the cold hemagglutination test and anti-streptococcus MG testing. Neither test is definitive, and more testing is required to confirm. Again, nothing is required of the patient other than a random venous blood sample for these tests (serum).

2. Rickettsial infections

Confirmation of the diagnosis generally necessitates further testing. Doctors are usually unable to determine if a patient has been infected with rickettsiae because conventional laboratory tests fail to identify these bacteria. Due to the rarity of normal access to these specialized blood tests, and the length of time it takes to conduct them, patients must be treated before test reports are obtained.

Useful Tests: (1) Blood tests that identify antibodies to rickettsiae (2) the removal of a small sample of skin for testing (biopsy) if they develop a rash. In the past, the complement fixation test was frequently utilized, however alternative tests are now employed to differentiate between immunoglobulin classes. As for the other procedures, the most popular are the immunoperoxidase assay and the enzyme-linked immunosorbent assay (ELISA). Microimmunofluorescence is the most popular of these assays.

3. Mononucleosis infectious

The heterophile agglutination test employs sheep RBCs, which do not typically react with human antibodies; when they do, and a high titer is indicated, mononucleosis is identified.

4. Mycotic infections

The same complement-fixation test may be used to identify fungal infections in deep tissues (such as the lungs).

5. Inflammatory conditions

The C-Reactive Protein Test (CRPA) is a serological test used to diagnose several inflammatory disorders. When there is tissue inflammation or necrosis, C-protein is secreted. When this C-protein and a certain antiserum are combined, a reaction occurs that results in a positive outcome. The degree of response is then rated from Plus 1 (1+) to Plus 4 (4+).

Diseases like these can have a beneficial impact:

a. Rheumatoid arthritis
b. Myocardial infarct
c. Certain malignant diseases

6. Rheumatoid arthritis

One test involves combining blood with small rubber (latex) beads coated with human antibodies. The latex beads stick together if Rheumatoid Factor (RF) is present. Rheumatoid arthritis can be diagnosed using this approach as a first-time screening test. The agglutination test involves the mixing of the blood being examined with red blood cells from a sheep that have been coated with rabbit antibodies. Blood cells congregate when RF is present. This is a common way to check for the presence of RF.

What Are the Different Types of Serology Tests and How Do They Work?

There are several serology tests available, all of them detect antibodies in a person's blood serum, which is its component and does not include red blood cells.

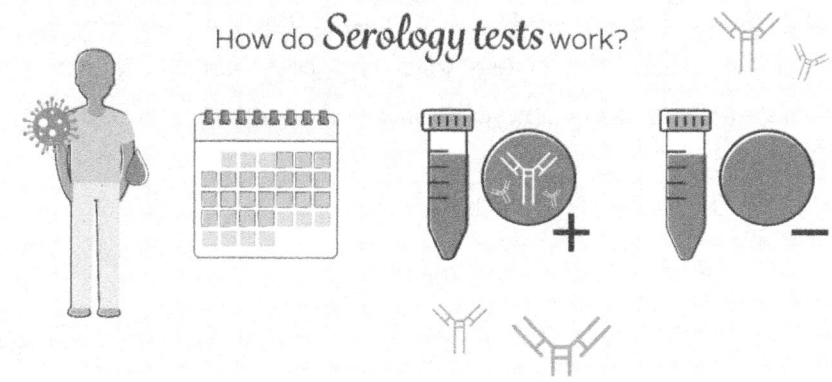

Qualitative serology tests offer a simple "yes" or "no" answer as to whether a person has been infected with SARS-CoV-2 in the past. Rapid serology tests, known as lateral flow assays (LFAs), are qualitative and produce a positive/negative result. This sort of test can determine a person's "serostatus," which is a word used in public health to identify whether a person is positive or negative for the antibodies of interest.

Quantitative serology procedures, like enzyme-linked immunosorbent assays (ELISAs) and chemiluminescent immunoassays (ChLIAs), offer more comprehensive results, such as antibody levels in a patient sample. Although knowing antibody levels is useful for research and has been used to assess whether a person is allowed to donate convalescent plasma, it is not required information for most people because it should not affect how they protect themselves and others against the virus. Indeed, many of the U.S. Food and Drug Administration's emergency use authorizations for quantitative serology tests typically state that they should only be used to offer patients with qualitative ("yes" or "no") replies.

SARS-COV-2 serology test accuracy and performance vary significantly; quantitative tests are typically more accurate than qualitative tests, owing to the comprehensive data collected.

What Types of Serology Testing Are Available?

Rapid serology test (RST)

This is a compact, portable, qualitative (positive or negative) lateral flow assay that may be performed at the point of care. Blood taken from a finger prick, saliva, or nasal swab fluid may be used in these assays. RSTs are frequently comparable to pregnancy tests in that the test displays colored lines to the user to indicate positive or negative findings. These tests most commonly look for patient antibodies (IgG and IgM) or viral antigens in the context of COVID-19. In certain situations, measuring baseline IgG and IgM titers (before infection) might be useful.

Enzyme-Linked immunosorbent assay (ELISA)

This is a laboratory-based test that can be qualitative or quantitative. Patients' whole blood, plasma, or serum samples are often used in these examinations. A plate coated with a viral protein of interest, such as Spike protein, is used in the test. The protein is then treated with patient samples, and if the patient has antibodies to the viral protein, they bond together. The coupled antibody-protein complex can then be identified using another antibody wash that produces a color or fluorescence readout. In the context of COVID-19, these tests are most commonly used to detect patient antibodies (IgM and IgG).

Neutralization assay

In a laboratory environment, this test depends on patient antibodies to inhibit viral infection of cells. Neutralization tests can inform researchers whether a patient has antibodies that are active and effective against the virus, even if the illness has previously been eradicated. These tests need the collection of whole blood, serum, or plasma from the patient. Cell culture, a laboratory-based method of cultivating cells that allow SARS-CoV-2 development, is used in neutralization tests (like VeroE6 cells). When viruses and cells are cultured in the presence of decreasing quantities of patient antibodies, researchers can see and measure how many antibodies in the patient serum are capable of preventing viral multiplication. This blocking effect can occur, for example, when the antibody binds to a key cell entrance protein on the virus.

Chemiluminescent immunoassay

A quantitative, laboratory-based diagnostic that uses whole blood, plasma, or serum samples from patients. A chemiluminescent microparticle immunoassay is a variant of this test that uses magnetic, protein-coated microparticles. The test involves combining patient samples with a known viral protein, buffer reagents, and particular enzyme-labeled antibodies, which enable a light-based, luminescent read-out. Any antibodies in the patient sample that respond to the viral protein will join together to create a complex. Then, (secondary) enzyme-labeled antibodies that bind to these complexes are added. This binding causes a chemical process that results in the production of light. The quantity of light emitted by each sample is then used to determine the number of antibodies present in a patient sample. This test may detect a variety of antibodies, including IgA, IgG, and IgM.

Serology Tests Are Classified into the Following Categories

Type of test	Time to results	What it tells us	Limitations
Rapid serology test	10 to 30 minutes	The existence or lack (qualitative) of anti-virus antibodies in patient serum.	The number of antibodies in the patient's serum, as well as whether these antibodies are capable of inhibiting virus growth.
Enzyme-linked immunosorbent assay (ELISA)	2 to 5 hours	The presence or absence (quantitative) of anti-virus antibodies in patient serum.	If the antibodies are capable of preventing virus proliferation.
Neutralization assay	3 to 5 days	Active antibodies present in patient serum that can block viral growth in a	Antibodies to viral proteins which are not involved in replication may be missed.

		cell culture system ex vivo.	
Chemiluminescent immunoassay	1 to 2 hours	The presence or absence (quantitative) of anti-virus antibodies in the patient serum.	If the antibodies are capable of preventing virus proliferation.

Chapter 7: Tumor Markers

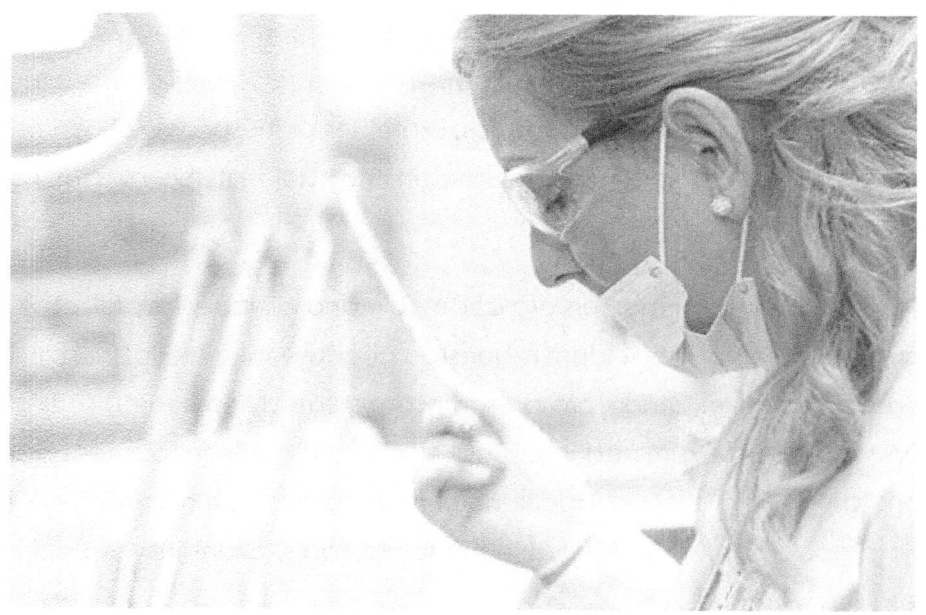

What Exactly Are Tumor Markers?

Tumor markers are substances, usually proteins, generated by cancer tissue or the body in reaction to the growth of cancer. Some of the substances are able to be detected in bodily fluids such as blood, urine, and tissues; therefore, these markers may be used in conjunction with other tests and procedures to identify and diagnose certain types of cancer, predict and monitor a person's response to certain treatments, and detect recurrence.

The concept of what defines a tumor marker has been widened lately. Newer assays that search for changes in genetic material (DNA, RNA) rather than proteins in patient samples have been developed. The genetic alterations have been linked to specific malignancies and can be utilized as tumor markers to help assess prognosis, direct focused treatment, and/or discover tumors at an early stage. Furthermore, technological advancements have resulted in tests that may analyze several genetic markers or marker panels at the same time, offering more information on tumor features. Examples of these, as well as more typical tumor markers, are provided in the table at the end of this section.

While several tumor markers are accessible and clinically helpful, others are available but are seldom requested because they are less sensitive and/or selective. Others are presently only utilized in research settings and are being examined in clinical studies. With continuous research and as the field evolves, additional tumor markers with higher efficacy will probably enter the market in the future years, eventually replacing less effective ones.

Limitations

While tumor marker tests can be quite informative, they have certain limitations:

- Many tumor markers may be increased in people with illnesses or diseases other than cancer.
- Some tumor markers are unique to a cancer single form, whilst others are seen in a variety of cancers.
- Not every person diagnosed with a certain cancer type will have an increased level of the matching tumor marker.
- Not all cancers have a tumor marker that has been identified as linked to them.

As a result, tumor markers are not diagnostic for cancer; nevertheless, for some forms of cancer, they give extra information that may be used in conjunction with a patient's medical history, physical exam, and other laboratory and/or imaging tests.

How are Tumor Markers Used?

Tumor markers can be utilized for several different purposes. Consequently, they are rarely used on their own. They can be used along with a tissue biopsy, bone marrow or blood smear test, and/or other tumor indicators, depending on the kind of malignancy. They are not conclusive, but they give extra information that can be useful:

Assist in the diagnosis
Tumor markers may be used to detect cancer and differentiate it from other illnesses with similar symptoms in a person who has symptoms.

Stage
If a person has cancer, tumor marker increases can assist identify whether cancer has spread (metastasized) to other tissues or organs and how far it has spread.

Screen

Most tumor markers are not sensitive or specific enough; therefore, they are not suitable for testing the general population; however, some may be used to screen for people who are at high-risk due to strong family history or specific risk factors for cancer.

Assist with therapy selection

A few tumor markers indicate which therapies may be helpful against a person's cancer. This is a developing field of study. More information may be found in the article "Genetic Tests for Targeted Cancer Therapy."

Ascertain the prognosis

Some tumor markers can be used to predict how aggressive a malignancy would be.

Track treatment success and detect recurrence

Tumor markers, particularly in advanced malignancies, can be utilized to evaluate therapy efficacy. If the marker level falls, the therapy is effective; if it remains elevated, modifications are required. (However, the information should be taken with caution because other diseases can occasionally cause tumor markers to rise or decline.). Along with directing therapy, one of the most significant applications for tumor markers is to monitor for cancer recurrence. If a tumor marker is raised before therapy, drops after treatment, and then begins to climb again over time, the cancer is likely to recur. If it stays elevated following surgery, likely, all of the malignancy has not been removed.

The table below contains examples of tumor markers that are used in each of these methods.

Table of Tumor Marker Examples

Tumor markers frequently have many functions and may be related to more than one form of cancer. This table contains tumor marker examples, as well as their many applications.

TUMOR MARKER	ASSOCIATED CANCER(S)	USUAL SAMPLE	USE(S)	COMMENTS
AFP (Alpha-fetoprotein)	Certain testicular, liver, ovarian.	Blood	Aids in diagnosis, treatment monitoring, and recurrence prevention.	Also increased during pregnancy and with hepatitis.
ALK gene rearrangements	Anaplastic large cell lymphoma, non-small cell lung cancer.	Tissue	Guides treatment.	Aids in the direction of focused therapy.
B-cell immunoglobulin gene rearrangement	B-cell lymphoma.	Bone marrow, tissue, body fluid, blood	Aids in the diagnosis, therapy monitoring, and recurrence prevention.	Identifies distinctive alterations in certain genes in B-cells.

Beta-2 microglobulin	Multiple myeloma, some leukemias, and lymphomas.	Blood, urine, CSF	Determines prognosis supervises treatment, and checks for recurrence.	Elevated in other diseases, such as kidney disease.
BCR-ABL	Chronic myeloid leukemia (CML) and BCR-ABL-positive acute lymphocytic leukemia (ALL).	Blood, bone marrow	Aids in diagnosis, treatment monitoring, and recurrence prevention.	
CA 15-3 (a Cancer antigen 15-3 & CA 27.29. Two different tests that are for the same marker	Breast.	Blood	Monitors treatment and recurrence.	Increased levels have also been discovered in several other cancers (lung, ovarian), benign breast diseases, endometriosis, and hepatitis.

CA 19-9 (Cancer antigen 19-9)	Pancreatic, sometimes bile ducts, gallbladder, stomach, colon.	Blood	Monitors treatment and recurrence.	In various kinds of digestive tract cancer, as well as non-cancerous conditions such as thyroid illness, pancreatitis, bile duct blockage, and inflammatory bowel disease, its levels are increased.
CA-125 (Cancer antigen 125)	Ovarian.	Blood	Help diagnose, monitors treatment, and for recurrence.	PID, uterine fibroids, endometriosis, and pregnancy, as well as the spread of other cancers (such as endometrial, peritoneal, and fallopian tubes).

Calcitonin	Medullary thyroid carcinoma (MTC) and C-cell hyperplasia.	Blood	Help diagnose, monitors treatment, and for recurrence.	Other cancers (lung, leukemias) are also increased; however, this test is not utilized to detect them.
CEA (Carcinoembryonic antigen)	Colon, breast, pancreatic, lung, ovarian, medullary thyroid, and others.	Blood	Cancer staging, prognosis, therapy, and recurrence monitoring.	Elevated in those with RA, hepatitis, COPD, colitis, pancreatitis, and cigarette smokers.
Chromogranin A (CgA)	Neuroendocrine tumors (carcinoid tumors, neuroblastoma).	Blood	Aids in diagnosis, treatment monitoring, and recurrence prevention.	For carcinoid tumors, it is one of the most sensitive tumor markers.

Marker	Cancer	Sample	Use	Notes
DCP (Des-gamma-carboxy prothrombin)	Hepatocellular carcinoma (HCC).	Blood	Monitors the treatment and detects any recurrence.	It can be used with an imaging study, AFP, AFP-L3%.
EGFR mutation	Non-small cell lung cancer and sometimes head and neck.	Tissue	Determines prognosis and also guides treatment.	Guides targeted therapies.
Estrogen and Progesterone receptors	Breast.	Tissue	Determines prognosis and also guides treatment.	Increased in hormone-dependent cancer.
Fibrin/Fibrinogen	Bladder.	Urine	Monitors the treatment and detects any recurrence.	

Gastrin	G-cell hyperplasia, gastrin-producing tumor (gastrinoma).	Blood	Help diagnose, monitors the treatment, and detects any recurrence.	Helps diagnose Zollinger-Ellison syndrome.
hCG (Human chorionic gonadotropin, also called Beta-hCG)	Testicular and trophoblastic disease, germ cell tumors, and choriocarcinoma.	Blood, urine	Help diagnose, monitors treatment, and for recurrence.	Elevated in pregnancy.
HER2	Breast, gastric, esophageal.	Tissue	Determines prognosis, guides treatment.	Helps with medicines that target HER2 receptors on cancer cells.

JAK2 mutation	Some types of leukemia, myeloproliferative neoplasms, especially polycythemia Vera.	Blood, bone marrow	Helps diagnose.	Detects gene mutations.
KRAS mutation	Colon, non-small cell lung cancer.	Tissue	Determines prognosis and also guides treatment.	Helps guide targeted therapies.
Lactate dehydrogenase (LD, LDH)	Testicular tumors and other germ cell tumors.	Blood	Guides and monitors treatment and recurrence.	Elevated in several diseases; may be utilized in various malignancies (e.g., lymphoma, melanoma, and neuroblastoma).

Monoclonal immunoglobulins	Multiple myeloma and Waldenstrom's macroglobulinemia.	Blood, urine	Aids in diagnosis, treatment monitoring, and recurrence prevention.	Detected by protein electrophoresis or serum-free light chains.
PSA (Prostate-specific antigen)	Prostate.	Blood	It can be utilized for screening, diagnosis, therapy monitoring, and recurrence prevention.	It is also increased in benign prostatic hyperplasia (BPH) and prostatitis; it might be utilized for screening.
SMRP (Soluble mesothelin-related peptides)	Mesothelioma (rare cancer associated with asbestos exposure).	Blood	Monitors treatment and recurrence.	It is frequently used in combination with imaging tests.

T-cell receptor gene rearrangement	T-cell lymphoma.	Bone marrow, tissue, body fluid, blood	Aids in diagnosis, treatment monitoring, and recurrence prevention.	Finds rearrangements in certain genes in T-cells.
Thyroglobulin	Thyroid.	Tissue and Blood	Reviews treatment and for recurrence.	After the thyroid is removed, it is used to evaluate its treatment.
Gene expression tests for Breast cancer (Such as Oncotype DX® and MammaPrint®)	Breast.	Tissue	Helps guide treatment and watches for recurrence.	Assess the likelihood of recurrence; help determine whether certain women with breast cancer can skip treatment.

Chapter 8: Testing for Body Fluid and Stool

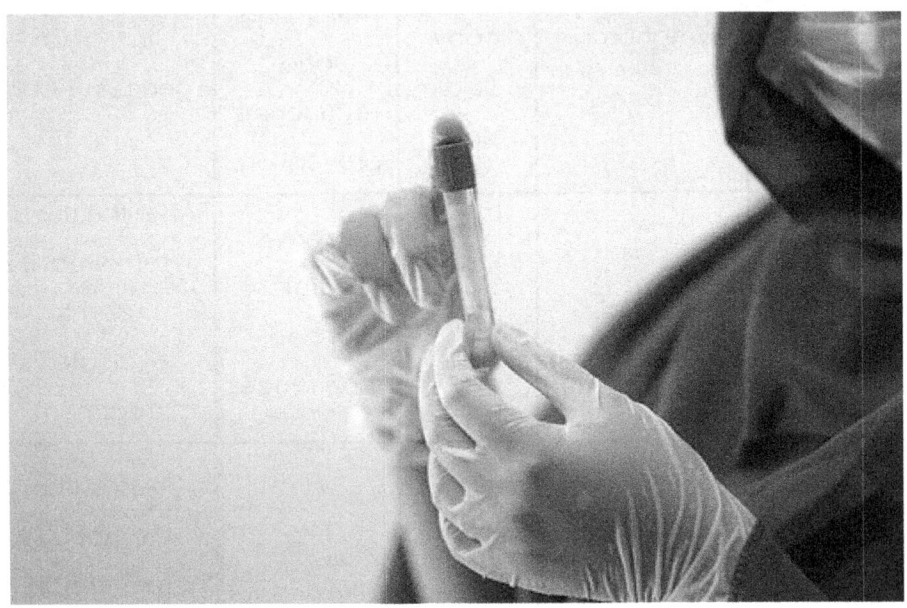

Clinical labs are getting an increasing number of requests to do regular testing on a wide range of bodily fluid types other than urine, serum, or plasma that have not been approved by assay producers. In many situations, the laboratory prefers these solicitations without taking into account the particular requirements of this type of testing. For a long time, laboratories have dissected these off-label sample types, and they have played an important role in detecting and treating a range of illnesses. In any event, the patient safety risk has not been fully recognized up to this time, and further regulatory requirements are adding another layer of complexity.

Clinical laboratories may now wonder if continuing to provide this service is worth the extra effort necessary to maintain administrative compliance. Regardless of the difficulties associated with off-label body fluid testing, it remains an excellent tool when it is used accurately and the risks are recognized and minimized. In addition to ensuring that the test execution characteristics are acceptable for the intended use, labs may increase patient security by collaborating with the clinical group to improve the appropriate use of the test and results interpretation.

What Exactly Are Off-Label Body Fluids?

Off-label bodily fluids refer to any liquid type that is not listed in the "Proposed Use" section of an item provided by the manufacturer of a Food and Drug Administration (FDA) approved method. They do not come from blood or urine and contain cerebrospinal fluid (CSF), serous fluids (peritoneal, pericardial, and pleural), synovial fluid, dialysis, and drainage fluids, among others. The neurotic buildup of these bodily fluids occurs as a result of a decreased rate or an enhanced generation of absorption. Every fluid type has an intriguing composition and, for the most part, is regarded as a critical sample because the collection is usually invasive.

What are the difficulties of off-label body fluid testing?

Until recently, off-label bodily fluid testing could be performed without the same stringent safeguards that are routinely applied to other in vitro diagnostics. Regulatory authorities have recently recognized the intriguing concept of each bodily fluid kind and the impact of these differences in chemical composition (electrolytes, proteins, lipids, pH, and so on.) may have on test execution. Currently, laboratories are obliged to analyze and record the presentation characteristics of each fluid type to ensure that it is suitable for the intended application.

Although some of the basic guidelines for urine and serum samples can be applied, several challenges when approving these off-label sample types remain, for example, gathering enough rare samples, verifying a wider scope of analyte fixations, finding an alternate technique for correlation, and evaluating reference interims.

Some other challenges are a lack of matrix-matched quality control materials, data on sample stability, and appropriate logical literature sources to develop clinical utility and reference ranges. Laboratories should fundamentally investigate the accessible restricted dispersed exams, since they may not be transferable to the lab's testing methods and patient populations.

Is there off-label body fluid testing guidance available?

There is little advice available for clinical labs. Although it is now compulsory to evaluate these tests, the validation amount is at the discretion of the laboratory director.

Clinical labs are moving in a limited way. Even though these updated tests are now required to be evaluated, the degree of approval is at the discretion of the laboratory executive. The College of American Pathologists (CAP) agendas are a good resource to ensure proper documentation for compliance. The most recent versions of the agendas have added regulatory requirements to implement the methodology, approve techniques, and report outcomes.

The Laboratory and Clinical Science Institute rules developed through the agreement method for the examination of bodily fluids are also essential resources. These archives are concerned with the clinical usefulness of analyte estimates in the majority of fluid types. They also advise clinical laboratories on results interpretation, reports, and analytical factors that affect body fluid estimates. A more recent widely disseminated survey paper by Block and Algeciras-Schimnich explicitly addresses serous fluids.

How Can Laboratories Lower Their Risk?

To reduce the risks associated with off-label bodily fluid testing, labs should first examine their existing test order volumes and patterns. They should conduct a rigorous audit to separate tests with established clinical usefulness, as depicted in the literature, from those that do not have. Tests that do not produce data that may be utilized to influence patient treatment or improve the clinical context in which they are ordered should stopped being put to use. To assist clinicians and patients in a better way, laboratories should focus their efforts on approving the most frequent fluid types and tests with well-established clinical value. Depending on the laboratory's size and the personnel amount, it may become more feasible to transmit low volume or even all off-label bodily fluid test requests to a reference laboratory.

Laboratories may also consider implementing approval processes to handle bodily fluid solicitations for those with dubious or limited usefulness or those that have not yet been fully approved. The Mayo Clinic method needs the laboratory director's authorization, and they just completed a similar procedure at University Hospitals Case Medical Center with their residents. They've authorized over 15 common scientific tests for use with a variety of off-label sample types.

For non-approved body liquid test requests, the on-call resident is responsible for reviewing the patient's restorative record and, if required, contacting the clinical group to understand why the test is sought and how the group intends to interpret the results. If the clinical utility is evident, we evaluate the measure's accuracy by running a dilution experiment to rule out matrix effects. If the dilution investigation findings satisfy our requirements, the resident likes the outcome's arrival.

Clinical laboratories must be aware of potential safety concerns throughout the testing procedure. It is their responsibility as laboratory specialists to support appropriate testing of off-label bodily fluids, ensure that the results presented are logically sound, and provide genuine results interpretation guidance — just as they would for blood, urine, and serum.

By expanding the test menu to include only clinically useful tests with appropriate interpretative data, labs can lower the risks associated with off-label testing while still providing clinicians with critical data for faster diagnosis and complicated patients' treatment.

The Purpose and Practicality of Body Fluid Validation and Testing

A broad range of neuropsychiatric diseases and treatments create unusual fluid buildup within the body. To determine the underlying cause of this buildup, clinicians often remove and localize fluid load, send fluid samples to clinical laboratories for investigation, and provide information on critical stages throughout the test method as part of the prognosis and evaluation process. In the past, laboratories used a variety of diagnostic methods to cross-examine these materials, such as counting and differentiating cells and biochemical analytes, as well as incubating cultures. Gathering a coordinated blood sample and selecting appropriate tests are also important aspects.

The Clinical and Laboratory Standards Institute (CLSI) is nearing completion of the second edition of the guideline paper, Body Fluid Analysis in Clinical Chemistry. This update covers topics across the whole testing procedure, providing laboratories with step-by-step instructions to examine the tests systematic presentation utilized to assess organically significant analytes in body fluid frameworks. Furthermore, this version will provide laboratories with a mechanism to distinguish and explore prior body fluid testing-related subtleties and difficulties.

The case discussion and research that accompany it provide a model not just of how clinicians use bodily fluid data to diagnose, manage, and treat patients, but also of the role of clinical laboratories in supporting patient care.

The Role of Laboratories in Patient Management

Clinical laboratories, as seen in this example, are important collaborators in giving notable results to patient treatment. In any event, laboratories are generally not responsible for collecting bodily fluids in the same manner that phlebotomists collect blood. Furthermore, as noted by most in vitro diagnostics manufacturers' intended use claims, bodily fluid testing is deemed an off-label usage of assays. According to regulatory and accrediting bodies, laboratories must undertake analytical approval for every test in which the sample type under investigation does not fall within the planned use statement. This creates a significant burden on laboratories to understand and manage pre-diagnostic circumstances linked to fluid assortment, as well as to authorize the display of any assays for which they plan to provide testing. Until now, the investigations that a laboratory may do to demonstrate appropriate execution on other matrices have not been extensively shown.

Transforming Body Fluid Challenges into Lessons Learned

Challenge 1

The fluid sort is determined by the location and source of the fluid collection as specified in the order structure. Because of the variety of components, laboratorians may not always have a clear understanding of the sample source. To begin with, the laboratory may have had limited, if any, input into the framework used to order body fluid tests; thus, these frames may include anatomic locations and fluid descriptions to recognize the emergence of fluids that do not coordinate the laboratory framework characterized sample sources, and explanation or interpretation is required. Frequently, laboratories receive bodily fluid samples labeled as drain fluid with minimal information other than the kind of drainage, such as "wound" or "Jackson Pratt," abbreviated as JP. The true location of assortment — sometimes a better hint to the fluid's identity — might be missing.

In the instance presented in this book, two samples arrived in the laboratory labeled with the specific anatomical location of the bodily fluid, "perihepatic and subhepatic." These specific fluid types were not permitted bodily fluid types, and all things considered, the technologist did consecutive dilutions to ensure that the chemical analytes demonstrated a direct response to rule out the presence of matrix blockage before discharging the findings. Interestingly, the sample labeled "right upper abdominal fluid" from channel 3 was examined undeniably for any further workup, since "abdominal" is a perceived synonym for peritoneal fluid, and was afterward considered as an acceptable source by this laboratory according to its usual working methods. Even though all of the samples were channel fluids from the patient's peritoneal cavity, the laboratory did successive dilutions on two of the three based on the descriptions supplied. This caused the lab's results to be delayed.

Lesson 1

Laboratories may choose not to examine bodily fluid types from non-approved locations and sources. However, to ensure effective patient treatment, they may need to call clinical teams for clarification. In our situation, the laboratory determined after a cursory inspection that the fluids in question originated in the patient's abdominal cavity and were most likely peritoneal fluid. Laboratories must decide whether to do additional accuracy tests on fluids labeled with anatomic description, as in our case, when the fluids are eventually shown to have originated from a location that has been authorized. The source and location are part of the doctor's instructions and should not be modified under any circumstances.

We suggest that laboratories collect data on bodily fluids submitted for testing. This will allow them to make sure that the fluid types as well as their source and location can be successfully allocated on the order, but also that they coordinate the laboratory's permitted bodily fluid test menu. The benefits of doing this for the laboratory is that it allows technicians to quickly determine if fluid is of an authorized type. The number of fluids that require inspection and perhaps needless work-up (solution, recuperation assessment) is determined by the ordering framework's accessible options.

Challenge 2

Isn't the body fluid matrix similar to plasma or serum? A bodily fluid matrix is made up of chemicals and molecules that include the analyte of interest. The analyte of interest is usually derived from blood filtered via circulation, which should reflect the plasma or serum structure. The quantities of electrolytes, proteins, and lipids in a bodily fluid can alter recovery and interfere with the precise estimate of analytes inside the body fluid matrix. The degree to which these molecules may interfere in a fluid matrix is fairly unclear and nearly impossible to anticipate in a fluid matrix, much like blood.

Lesson 2

Interference evaluations are critical components of diagnostic body fluid approval that aim to ensure the accuracy of reported body fluid results. Recuperation tests promote understanding of how interference affects accuracy. Making a succession of bodily fluid aliquots with increasing centralizations of an interferer that are contrasted with the findings from an unaffected sample can be used to lead studies. In addition, laboratories should carefully consider using visual or spectrophotometric evaluation of bodily fluid by a computerized device to determine the interference concentration. In the case I describe in this book, the laboratory noticed that the fluid from channel

1 was dark-colored, maybe due to developed blood buildup in the hepatic fluid pocket or the presence of bile. Laboratories should have a plan in place for how to handle reports when hemolysis (hemoglobin) or icterus (bilirubin) limits are exceeded. Some choices include canceling the test, noting the outcome with a note, or attempting to dilute the interference to report a result.

Challenge 3

Laboratories lack control over a variety of bodily fluids, which has several repercussions. Because of the fairly diverse range of providers that collect bodily fluids and other samples, the fluid volume and container sent to the laboratory are likely to differ. It's worth noting what it may be named (see Challenge and Lesson 1).

Lesson 3

The containers used to transport samples to the laboratory and the bodily fluid quantities given may be an instant reflection of minimal fluid burden, what the restorative group can obtain, or a lack of information from the laboratory on the basic volume necessary for testing. Laboratories' discussions and active interaction with suppliers in charge of collecting non-blood samples would be wise to include a list of appropriate collection containers, in addition to the laboratory's volume and data requirements for body fluid samples. It is important to share this information to get the volume required to complete bodily fluid tests. Furthermore, samples delivery in a suitable container ensures that the test will not be canceled because it cannot be completed as received.

Challenge 4

Which tests are beneficial and should be approved? Because these fluid tests are considered routine in an analytic evaluation, physicians expect findings to be returned quickly for patient treatment. The fluid cell count is a fantastic model, since it can be used to detect malignant or infectious causes of fluid buildup. Regardless, bilirubin was seldom calculated in the scenario described in this chapter, despite concerns about probable bile leakage.

Lesson 4

Some biochemical analytes are helpful in some bodily fluids, whereas others have not. When we looked into our provided case, we found that all fluids had enlarged total nucleated cells with a preponderance of neutrophils, which was suggestive of illness. Extra biochemical tests in support of a compelling etiology found decreased glucose concentrations and pH; nevertheless, the precise choice point for an aberrant proportion of glucose from fluid to plasma isn't well defined, and pH has a proven value only when assessed in pleural fluids for this reason. These biochemical evaluations were likely of little importance, and in this case, the cell tally was the most useful for a diagnosis.

In our personal case, there was early suspicion of a bile leak. Interestingly, clinicians did not order bilirubin tests, maybe due to the unpleasant look of the fluid and the patient's prior medical history. The ERCP procedure used on the patient's following ED visit did confirm a bile leak. Lipid analysis in peritoneal fluids distinguishes between dangerous and non-harmful causes; nevertheless, its evaluation of a serious-looking fluid (channel 3) was likely futile in this circumstance.

Remember that bodily fluid values are best translated in conjunction with contemporaneous estimation in serum. In our situation, for example, amylase was calculated several times without coordinated blood collection. Amylase fluid to blood proportions provides greater interpretative information when seeking to distinguish pancreatic origin fluid. Normally, total protein and LDH are also measured along with bodily fluids. This is done frequently to classify the fluid as an exudate; nevertheless, the Light's Criteria application is better reserved for symptomatic evaluation of pleural liquids. Because this fluid originated in the patient's peritoneum in our model, it may have been increasingly appropriate to first assess the serum-ascites fluid albumin gradient.

Creating an appropriate test menu and approval process allows laboratories to confidently offer a body fluid test menu to meet clinical demands. Clinical laboratories should be aware of the whole testing process and provide tools that primarily assess the clinical applicability and usability of analyte estimates in bodily fluids. After the release of the second edition of CLSI's rule, and Body Fluid Analysis in Clinical Chemistry, laboratories will be able to start a body fluid approval project to check an assay's performance on body fluid clinical usefulness and testing menu matrices.

Chapter 9: Arterial Blood Gas Analysis

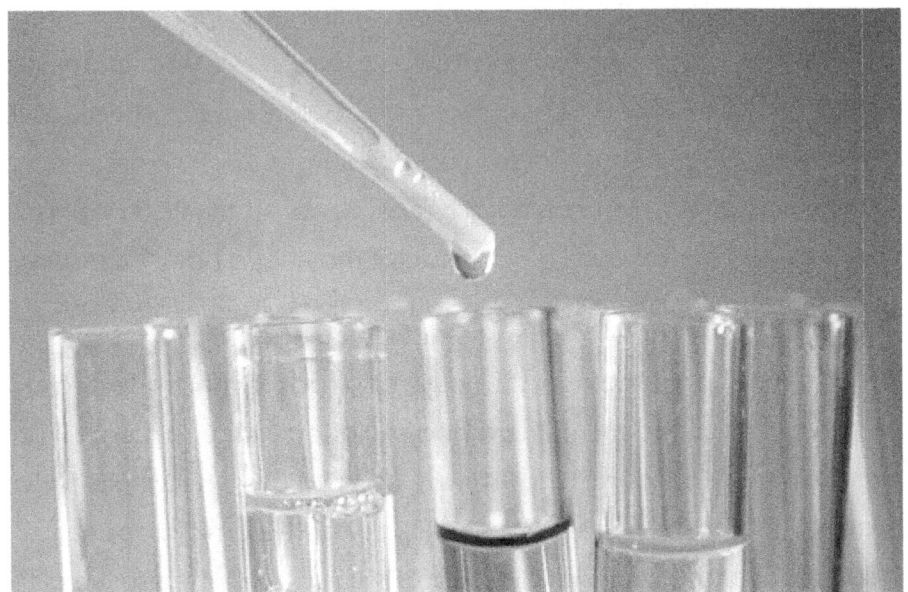

The Arterial Blood Gas (ABG) analysis method and checking is a fundamental component in the management and diagnosis of the oxygenation status and corrosive base equalization of high-risk patients, as well as in the care of essentially unwell patients in the Intensive Care Unit. Both areas exhibit rapid and life-threatening alterations in all systems involved, any doctor, including anesthesiologists, must have a thorough understanding of the corrosive base balance. However, understanding ABGs and their interpretation can be highly perplexing and time-consuming in some situations. There are several techniques in the literature to direct the ABGs interpretation. The presentation in this chapter does not include all of those approaches, such as base abundance analysis or Stewart's solid ion contrast, but a cohesive and ordered methodology is demonstrated to allow us to make a much easier interpretation via them. The best possible use of the concepts of corrosive base balance will assist the medical services provider not only to follow a patient's development but also to assess the feasibility of the treatment being provided.

ABG study is a fundamental component in the management and diagnosis of a patient's oxygenation status and corrosive base balance. The effectiveness of this diagnostic equipment is contingent on the ability to correctly interpret the results. Corrosive base balance disorders can cause complications in a variety of illness conditions, and the deviation from the norm can occasionally be so great that it becomes a life-threatening risk factor. Any clinician, including intensivists and anesthesiologists, must have a thorough understanding of corrosive base balance.

The three most often used methods for dealing with corrosive base physiology are the HCO3 (about pCO2), standard base excess (SBE), and solid ion difference (SID). Stewart's notion of SID, which is defined as the complete contrast between fully separated anions and cations, has been around for a long time. The weak acids and CO2 balance this distinction, as stated by the electrical neutrality law. Because SID is defined in terms of weak acids and CO2, it has been renamed effective SID (SIDe), which is indistinguishable from "bugger base." Similarly, Stewart's unique word for total feeble acid concentration (ATOT) is now defined as the dissociated (A-) plus undissociated (AH) weak acid structures. When ordinary concentration is caused by A-, this is naturally known as the anion gap (AG). As a result, when all 3 methods are used to evaluate the acid-base status of a particular blood test, the results are virtually identical.

Blood Gas Test

A blood gas test determines the carbon dioxide and oxygen concentrations in someone's blood. It can also be used to determine the blood pH, or how acidic it is. The test is commonly referred to as a blood gas examination or an arterial blood gas (ABG) test.

Red blood cells transport carbon dioxide and oxygen and move them throughout your body and are called blood gases.

Oxygen goes in the blood and carbon dioxide leaves as blood moves through the lungs. A blood gas test is used to see how efficiently your lungs transport oxygen into your blood and expel carbon dioxide from it.

Imbalances in your blood's carbon dioxide, oxygen, and pH levels can indicate the existence of certain diseases. These might include:

- Heart failure
- Kidney failure
- Uncontrolled diabetes
- Chemical toxicity
- Narcotics overdose
- Hemorrhage
- Shock

When you have symptoms of any of these diseases, your primary care physician may order a blood gas test. The test requires the collection of a little amount of blood from a vein. It's a safe and simple approach that just takes a few minutes to complete.

Why Is a Blood Gas Test Performed?

A blood gas test determines the exact amounts of carbon dioxide and oxygen in your body. This allows your primary care physician to assess how well your kidneys and lungs are working.

This is a test commonly used in medical clinics to identify how to care for critically ill patients. It does not play a significant role in primary care, although it may be used in a pneumonic function clinic or laboratory.

If you have symptoms of a carbon dioxide, oxygen, or pH imbalance, your doctor may order a blood gas test. Among the symptoms are:

- Confusion
- Breathing difficulties
- Nausea

These symptoms might be signs of a variety of illnesses, including asthma and chronic obstructive pulmonary disease (COPD).

If your primary care physician suspects you are suffering from any of the following disorders, he or she may conduct a blood gas test:

- Renal failure
- Metabolic disorder
- Lung disease
- Injuries to the neck or head impair breathing

Distinguishing abnormalities in pH and blood gas levels can also help your primary care physician screen treatment for specific illnesses, such as lung and renal ailments.

A blood gas test is frequently done along with other procedures, such as a blood glucose test to monitor blood sugar levels and a creatinine blood test to evaluate kidney function.

What Are the Risks Associated with a Blood Gas Test?

A blood gas test is considered a generally safe procedure, since it does not require a large sample of blood.

Regardless, you should always inform your doctor about any current medical problems that may cause you to bleed more than usual. You should also inform them if you are using any over-the-counter or prescribed medications, such as blood thinners, that may affect your bleeding.

The following are possible symptoms associated with a blood gas test:

- Experiencing dizziness.
- The buildup of blood under the skin.
- Bruises or bleeding at the puncture location.
- Infection at the site of the puncture.

Inform your primary care physician if you have any unexpected or delayed symptoms.

How does a blood gas test work?

A blood gas test starts with the gathering of a small sample of blood. Arterial blood can be drawn from an artery in your arm, wrist, or groin, as well as from a prior artery line if you are currently hospitalized. A blood gas test can also be venous, requiring a little prick to the heel from a vein capillary or an existing IV.

A healthcare provider will first disinfect the infusion site with a germicide. When they find an artery, doctors inject a needle into it and take blood. When the needle is inserted, you may feel a little prick. Because of arteries have more smooth muscle layers than veins, some people believe that a blood gas test from an artery is more difficult than drawing blood from a vein.

After the needle has been removed, the expert will apply pressure for a few minutes before applying a bandage to the cut damage.

The blood test will then be dissected using a versatile machine or in an on-site laboratory. To provide an accurate test result, the sample must be examined within 10 minutes after the procedure.

Explaining The Result of a Blood Gas Test

The findings of a blood gas test can help your primary care physician evaluate different illnesses or determine how effective therapies are working for certain diseases, such as lung disease. It also indicates if your body is compensating for the imbalance.

Because of the possibility of compensating for certain qualities, which will result in the correction of other values/qualities, the person to read the results must be a qualified healthcare provider with expertise in blood gas elucidation.

The test assesses:

Arterial blood pH

It measures the concentration of hydrogen ions in the blood. A pH less than 7.0 is considered acidic, whereas a pH more than 7.0 is considered alkaline or basic. A lower blood pH can show that your blood is becoming more acidic and contains more carbon dioxide. A higher blood pH might indicate that your blood is becoming more basic and has a greater bicarbonate content.

Bicarbonate
It is a synthetic that keeps the blood pH from being either acidic or too basic.

Partial oxygen pressure

It is a percentage of the dissolved oxygen pressure in the blood. It governs how effectively oxygen can diffuse from the lungs into the blood.

Carbon dioxide partial pressure

It is a proportion of the dissolved carbon dioxide pressure in the blood. It governs how effectively carbon dioxide may leave the body.

Oxygen saturation
It is a percentage of the amount of oxygen carried by the hemoglobin in red blood cells.

Generally, values are:

- Arterial blood ph: 7.38 to 7.42
- Incomplete pressure of oxygen: 75 to 100 mm Hg
- Incomplete pressure of carbon dioxide: 38 to 42 mm Hg
- Bicarbonate: 22 to 28 milliequivalents per liter
- Oxygen saturation: 94 to 100%

If you reside above sea level, your blood oxygen levels may be lower.

If the data are from a capillary, venous, or sample, they will have an unusual reference range.

Chapter 10: Renal Function Tests

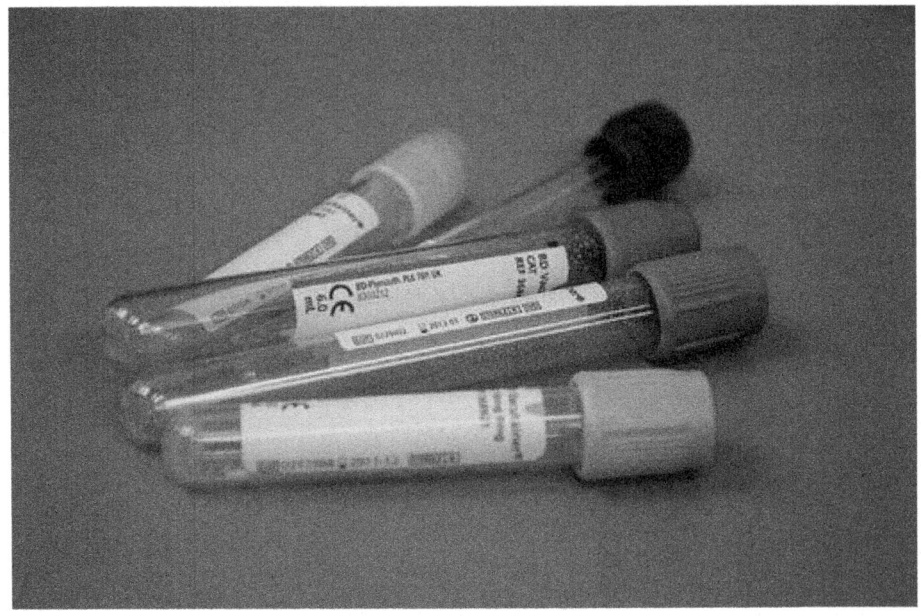

The kidneys play an important role in the elimination of waste and toxins such as urea, uric acid, and creatinine, as well as in the regulation of extracellular fluid volume, electrolyte concentrations, and serum osmolality, besides in the production of the hormones such as erythropoietin, renin, and 1,25 dihydroxy vitamin D. The nephron is the functional unit of the kidney, consisting of the proximal, glomerulus, and distal tubules, as well as the collecting duct. Renal function evaluation is important in the management of individuals with kidney disease or diseases affecting renal capacity. Renal capacity tests are useful in identifying the renal infection existence, monitoring the kidneys' response to therapy, and determining renal illness development. According to the National Institutes of Health, chronic kidney disease

(CKD) affects around 14% of the population. Diabetes and hypertension are the most well-known causes of CKD worldwide.

This chapter provides information on the most essential biochemical assays for assessing renal function.

Specimen Collection

Specimen collection requirements are determined by the technique or test sought. A random blood sample is sufficient for serum creatinine and blood urea nitrogen (BUN) values, as no further arrangements are necessary for the patient. Regardless, recent high protein consumption may have a significant influence on blood creatinine and urea levels. Similarly, hydration states can have a substantial impact on BUN estimates.

For urine collections over time, for example, the 24-hour pee creatinine clearance, it is critical that pee be collected accurately during the required time range, since under or over collection will impact conclusive findings. As a result, a coordinated collection lasting 5 to 8 hours is preferable to a collection that lasts 24 hours.

Midstream urine must be collected for urine testing because it is less likely to be contaminated by epithelial cells and commensal microscopic organisms.

Procedures

Renal function assessment

Several clinical laboratory tests may be used to investigate and evaluate kidney function. Clinically, the most practical methods to evaluate renal function are to look for proteinuria (albuminuria) and calculate the glomerular filtration rate (GFR).

Glomerular filtration rate

The glomerular filtration rate is the best indicator of glomerular capacity (GFR).

A normal GFR for an adult male is around 90 to 120 ml per minute. GFR is found by the rate in milliliters per minute at which compounds in plasma are separated through the glomerulus or the amount of a material that can be removed from the blood. The following are the characteristics of a perfect GFR marker:

- It should appear internally in the plasma at a consistent rate.
- It should be freely filtered into the glomerulus.
- It should not be reabsorbed or discharged by the renal tubule.
- It should not experience extra-renal elimination.

Because there is no such endogenous marker at the moment, exogenous GFR markers are used. GFR assessment using inulin, a polysaccharide, is regarded as the gold standard for GFR assessment. It consists of inulin infusion followed by blood level measurement after a predetermined interval to evaluate the inulin clearance rate. Radioisotopes, such as technetium-99 labeled diethylene-triamine-pentaacetate (99 Tc-DTPA) and chromium-51 ethylene-diamine-tetra-

acidic corrosive, are also used as exogenous markers (51 Cr-EDTA). Iohexol, a non-radioactive differentiation specialist, is the most promising exogenous marker, particularly in children.

The discomfort associated with the use of exogenous markers, namely that testing must be conducted at particular facilities, and the difficulties in detecting these chemicals, has enabled the use of endogenous markers.

Creatinine

Creatinine is the most often used endogenous measure to assess glomerular capacity. The measured creatinine clearance is used as an indication of GFR. This entails collecting urine over 24 hours, or ideally over a carefully coordinated span of 5 to 8 hours because 24-hour collections are notoriously inconclusive.

The equation is then used to calculate creatinine freedom:

$$C = (U \times V)/P$$

U = urinary concentration, C = clearance, P = plasma concentration, and V = urinary flow rate (volume/time e.g., ml/min).

Creatinine clearance should be modified to take into account body surface area. Incomplete or incorrect urine collection is one of the major factors impacting the accuracy of this test; thus, the scheduled collection is advantageous. Furthermore, due to tubular discharge, creatinine overestimates GFR by 10% to 20%.

Creatinine is produced by the body at a constant pace as a result of creatine phosphate in muscle. In most cases, the kidney fully removes creatinine from the blood. A decrease in renal clearance results in an increase in blood creatinine. The measurement of creatinine levels daily is based on muscle mass, so there is a difference in creatinine levels between females and males with lower creatinine values in children and individuals with decreased muscle mass. Diet also affects creatinine levels. These levels might rise by up to 30% after consuming red meat. Lower creatinine levels are observed in pregnancy when GFR increases. Furthermore, serum creatinine is a later indication of renal impairment — renal capacity is reduced by 50% before serum creatinine rises.

Serum creatinine is also utilized in GFR evaluation models such as the CKD-EPI equation and the Modified Diet in Renal Disease equation (MDRD). The eGFR equations are better than serum creatinine alone since they take into account age, race, and gender. GFR is classified into the following phases based on the severity of the kidney disease.

Improving Global Outcomes (KDIGO) chronic kidney disease (CKD) phases:

- Stage 1 GFR values higher than 90 ml/min/1.73 m
- Stage 2 GFR values from 60 to 89 ml/min/1.73 m
- Stage 3a GFR values from 45 to 59 ml/min/1.73 m
- Stage 3b GFR values from 30 to 44 ml/min/1.73 m
- Stage 4 GFR values from 15 to 29 ml/min/1.73 m
- Stage 5 GFR smaller values than 15 ml/min/1.73 m (for renal disease in its end-stage)

These provide a more straightforward estimate of GFR without the urine collection or the use of foreign materials. However, because they employ serum creatinine, they are also impacted by the problems surrounding serum creatinine estimation, and therefore the adjustment for gender, race, and age.

Blood Urea Nitrogen (BUN)

Urea or BUN is a nitrogen-containing compound that is formed in the liver as a result of protein digestion in the urea cycle. The kidneys remove around 85% of urea; the remainder is excreted through the gastrointestinal (GI) tract. Serum urea levels rise when renal clearance is reduced (as in acute and chronic renal impairment/failure). Urea levels may also rise in situations other than a renal disease, such as upper GI hemorrhage, catabolic states, dehydration, and high protein diets. Urea levels may be reduced by fasting, a low-protein diet, and severe liver disease. Serum creatinine is a more accurate measure of renal capacity than urea; nevertheless, urea is increased before the renal illness.

BUN proportion

When the BUN is elevated, creatinine can assist distinguish between pre-renal and renal causes. The proportion is close to 20:1 in pre-renal illness, whereas it is closer to 10:1 in intrinsic renal ailment.

Cystatin C

It is a protein with a low subatomic weight that acts as a protease inhibitor and is produced by every nucleated cell in the body. It is formed at a constant pace and is completely filtered by the kidneys. Cystatin C levels in the blood are inversely related to glomerular filtration rate (GFR). In other words, high numbers indicate low GFRs, whereas low values indicate greater GFRs, such as creatinine. Cystatin C's renal therapy differs from creatinine. While both are completely filtered by glomeruli, unlike creatinine, cystatin C is reabsorbed and utilized by proximal renal tubules after separation. As a result, under normal settings, cystatin C does not penetrate the final expelled urine in significant quantities. Cystatin C levels are measured in both serum and urine. Cystatin C advantages over creatinine include that it is unaffected by age, muscle mass, or nutrition, and several studies have demonstrated that it is a more reliable measure of GFR than creatinine, particularly in early renal failure. Cystatin C has also been included in eGFR calculations, such as the combined creatinine-cystatin KDIGO CKD-EPI equation.

Thyroid illness, cancer, and smoking may all affect Cystatin C levels:

Albuminuria and proteinuria

Albuminuria refers to the presence of 30 to 300 mg of albumin in the urine daily. Because there is no such biological atom as microalbumin, the phrase is now simply referred to as urine albumin. Albuminuria is used to diagnose early nephropathy in diabetics; it is an independent diagnostic for the cardiovascular disease since it indicates increased endothelial porousness and is also a sign of chronic renal impairment. Urine albumin can be calculated as an albumin/creatinine ratio in 24-hour pee samples or early morning/random samples. The albuminuria occurrence on 2 occasions when urine contamination is prohibited indicates glomerular dysfunction. The albuminuria occurrence for at least 3 months is indicative of chronic kidney disease. Proteinuria is defined as consuming more than 300 mg of protein per day. Every day, up to 150 mg of protein might be found in urine (30% globulins; 30% globulins; 40% Tamm Horsfall protein).

Protein levels in urine may have increased as a result of:

Glomerular proteinuria

This is caused by abnormalities in the glomerular filtration boundary's perm selectivity to plasma proteins (e.g., nephrotic or glomerulonephritis disorder)

Tubular proteinuria

This is caused by insufficient protein cylindrical reabsorption (e.g., interstitial nephritis)

Overflow proteinuria

This is caused by increased protein concentrations in the plasma (e.g., various myoglobinuria, myeloma-Bence Jones protein)

Irritation or tumor of the urinary tract

Urine protein can be measured using either a 24-hour urine collection or an irregular urine protein: creatinine ratio (early morning test-like and progressively illustrative of the 24-hour test).

The KDIGO classification distinguishes 3 stages of albuminuria:

- A1: Creatinine concentration of less than 30 mg/g
- A2: creatinine concentrations ranging from 30 to 300 mg/g
- A3: Creatinine concentrations more than 300 mg/g

Urine protein discharge in nephrotic syndrome exceeds 3.5 g per day and is associated with edema, hypercholesterolemia, and hypoalbuminemia.

Tubular Function Tests

The renal tubules have an important role in the reabsorption of electrolytes, water, and acid-base balance maintenance. Electrolytes, potassium, chloride, sodium, magnesium, and phosphate can all be measured in urine in the same way as glucose can. The estimation of urine osmolality takes into account the concentrating capacity of urine tubules. A urine osmolality of more than 750 mOsmol/Kg H_2O indicates that tubules have a normal concentrating capability. To rule out nephrogenic diabetes insipidus, a water deprivation test might be used. Similarly, an ammonium chloride test can be used to confirm the diagnosis of distal renal tubular acidosis (dRTA) with the failure to ferment urine to a pH less than 5.3. There is aminoaciduria, phosphaturia, glycosuria, and bicarbonate loss in Fanconi's disease (proximal RTA).

Urine Examination

Urine analysis encompasses physical perception, microscopic, and chemical examination of urine characteristics to aid in disease diagnosis. Evaluating clarity and color are examples of physical perception. Pee is typically straw-colored, but in the presence of dehydration, urine takes on a darker color. Red urine may indicate porphyria or hematuria, or it may be the result of dietary intake of nutrients such as beets. Because of urinary tract pollution, cloudy urine may be observed in the presence of pyuria. Explicit gravity, which is a measure of renal concentrating capacity, may be determined using a urine dipstick and chemical or refractometry. The healthy range for explicit gravity is 1.003 to 1.030, which increases with concentrated urine and decreases with dilute one.

Urine dipsticks use chemical analysis to provide a subjective assessment of different analytes in urine.

Dipstick employs dry chemical techniques to detect the presence of protein, blood, ketones, glucose, bilirubin, nitrite, urobilinogen, and leukocyte esterase. These might be followed by a point-of-care test near a patient. Color changes that occur as a result of the urine interaction with the chemicals on the paper of the dipstick are evaluated compared to the color graph manual for the interpretation of the results.

Analytes measured on urine dipstick protein should not be detected in routine urine samples. In normal urine, bilirubin is not found. Glucose is not detectable in healthy people, but it may be recognized in diabetes mellitus, renal glycosuria, and pregnancy when the renal edge of 180 mg/dl is reduced. The presence of ascorbic acid, often known as vitamin C, and a few antibiotics may affect the outcomes. After renal tract injury or contamination, blood may be accessible, with ascorbic acid having a deleterious effect. Urine dipstick differentiates the globin portion of hemoglobin and, as a result, cannot detect the presence of hemoglobin or myoglobin in the urine. In addition, hemoglobinuria and immaculate red blood cells (RBC) are seen. RBC per high-power field in normal urine ranges from 0 to 3 while white blood cells (WBC) range from 0 to 5. Ketones can be obtained when fasting, in diabetic ketoacidosis, or during acute vomiting. The ketone beta-hydroxybutyrate is not detected by the urine dipstick, only acetoacetate and CH3)2CO (acetone). Bilirubin is identified in the presence of conjugated hyperbilirubinemia, and urobilinogen may be present regularly; however, it is absent in the presence of conjugated hyperbilirubinemia and increased in the presence of hemolysis and prehepatic jaundice. Nitrite and leukocyte esterase are indicators of urinary tract illness. Some microorganisms, such as Enterobacteriaceae, convert nitrates to nitrites.

Wet-prep urine analysis is used to determine the presence of cells, crystals, casts, and microorganisms. Red blood cell casts are often associated with glomerulonephritis, whereas white ones are associated with pyelonephritis. WBC casts and white blood cells indicate contamination/infection; red blood cells suggest renal injury, and RBC casts imply cylindrical harm or glomerulonephritis. Protein-containing hyaline casts can occur in glomerular disease. **Crystals can also be seen in urine and are indicative of the following conditions:**

- Pseudogout is characterized by rectangular triple phosphate crystals.
- Uric corrosive crystals are needle-shaped and associated with gout.
- Oxalate crystals are envelope-formed and can be used to treat ethylene glycol toxicity or secondary and primary hyperoxaluria.
- Cystine crystals are hexagonal, as seen in cystinuria.

A recently voided midstream urine sample is the best for urine inquiry or analysis. Because it is less likely to be contaminated by commensal microscopic organisms and epithelial cells, midstream urine is utilized.

Acute Renal Impairment Vs. Chronic Renal Impairment

Acute renal impairment, also known as acute kidney injury, refers to the sudden onset of kidney damage within a few hours or days. Chronic kidney illness/disease is caused by long-term diseases, such as diabetes and hypertension. **Acute kidney injury can be caused by any of the following factors:**

- Causes of decreased blood flow to the kidneys (pre-renal causes), such as cardiogenic and hypotensive shock, dehydration, and blood loss following severe injury.
- Causes that induce direct kidney injuries (intrinsic/renal causes), such as nephrotoxic prescriptions and other toxins,

sepsis, malignancies such as myeloma, immune system illness, or diseases that cause damage to the kidney tubules or inflammation.
- Causes of urinary tract obstruction, such as bladder, cervical malignant development, or prostate, massive kidney stones, and blood clusters in the urine system.

It should be noted that pre-renal kidney injury might progress to acute tubular necrosis (ATN) and induce intrinsic renal damage.

Urine yield is a good tool for measuring kidney function and is used in rules to determine (AKI). Patients with AKI have oliguria (under 400 ml for each day). RIFLE (injury, risk, loss of kidney function, failure, and end-stage kidney infection) categorization is based on serum creatinine, GFR alterations, and urine yield determinants. The Acute Kidney Injury Network (AKIN) characterization criteria for AKI also include serum creatinine changes and urine yield; however, it does not rely on GFR changes and does not require a baseline serum creatinine.

Other laboratory tests, in addition to serum creatinine, play an important role in the diagnosis of AKI and aid in distinguishing between different types of acute kidney injury. This is essential because it will dictate the correct administration to the patient, patients with pre-renal causes will receive a fluid replacement and those with renal and post-renal reasons will receive more minimum fluids.

The estimation of extended urine explicit gravity (greater than 1.020) in dehydration and pre-renal cases is one of the tests that may assist in determining if the renal damage is pre-renal, renal, or post-renal. Under light microscopy, the presence of red and white blood cells, casts, tubular epithelial, or crystals in the urine residual might assist in the differential diagnosis.

Fractional excretion of sodium (FeNa) can assist differentiate acute tubular necrosis from pre-renal uremia. It requires the determination of serum creatinine and salt levels, as well as the determination of creatinine and sodium levels in spot urine samples. The fractional excretion is calculated using the following equation: FeNa = 100 × (urine sodium x serum creatinine) / (serum sodium x urinary creatinine). A score less than 1% indicates pre-renal levels, whereas a value of more than 2% indicates intrinsic causes. Nonetheless, the FeNa is unreliable in diuretic-treated individuals. Spot urine sodium convergences of less than 20 mmol/l are indicative of pre-renal AKI. The fractional excretion of urea measured according to FeNa using blood urea and urine urea rather than sodium can also be used to distinguish between pre-renal and intrinsic AKI, with values less than 35% indicating pre-renal impairment. A urine osmolality of more than 500 mOsm/kg is associated with pre-renal causes, whereas a serum osmolality (about 300 mOsm/kg) is associated with an intrinsic cause.

Novel Biomarkers

A few novel biomarkers are useful in determining AKI and in differentiating between stable CKD and AKI, as well as pre-renal and intrinsic AKI. These include low-atomic weight proteins found in the systemic circulation and subject to glomerular filtration (for example, cystatin C, retinol restricting protein, and beta2-microglobulin) and proteins produced in response to cell/tissue damage (NGAL, kidney injury molecule 1 (KIM-1), L-type fatty acid-binding protein (L-FABP), beta-trace protein, and FGF23). With further research, its optimal clinical value will be recognized.

Indications

The indications for evaluating renal capacity span from acute emergency to chronic situations. Renal capacity tests are primarily used to diagnose renal illness, establish optimal patient administration, and avoid future worsening of renal function. Other indications in patients who have been diagnosed with a renal malady are to stage the degree or type of renal ailment, monitor the course of renal ailment to ensure that optimal administration occurs on time, and monitor the response to medications. In other cases, renal capacity tests may be necessary to develop and screen renal capacity before starting a known or possibly nephrotoxic therapeutic substance for patient treatment. Renal function tests are also recommended in transplant contributors to assess the original benefactor suitability and identify any substantial decline in renal function post-donation. A renal capacity test can also be performed to determine whether part of the kidney's capacity unit (nephron) is impacted, such as glomerular or tubular illness.

Potential diagnosis

Renal capacity tests can be used to assess total renal capacity by direct estimate or measurement of the glomerular filtration rate. GFR estimation is used to assess the existence of renal debilitation and can identify the stage and presence of chronic kidney illness/disease when lowered over a predefined period. Furthermore, renal capacity tests can be performed to assess whether kidney disease is chronic or acute.

In the case of urine albumin, it might be used to detect nascent nephropathy in high-risk individuals such as diabetics.

Tubular capacity disorders, such as Fanconi syndrome, can be identified using renal capacity tests, especially the estimation of glucose, urinary amino acids, phosphate, and pH.

Normal and critical finding

A healthy adult guy has a GFR of 90 to 120 ml per minute. A GFR measured to be less than 15 ml per minute is associated with end-stage renal failure, requiring renal replacement therapy, such as dialysis. The existence of a normal GFR does not rule out the possibility of kidney infection, which can be verified by proteinuria/albuminuria or imaging.

The reference intermediates for serum creatinine and urea are gender and age-dependent.

The presence of electrolytes in urine is dependent on the duration of hydration, the status of urine collection separated from neurotic variables, and reference intervals are frequently broad and dependent on the clinical context.

Internal Factors

Creatinine

Preanalytical issues like high-protein intake and more muscle mass, might result in high creatinine values that are not indicative of a person's true renal capacity. Similarly, serum creatinine as a measure of renal capacity is usually inconclusive in persons with reduced muscle mass, such as the elderly, amputees, and people affected by muscular dystrophy. Creatinine is often measured using an automated analyzer and either a colorimetric reaction is known as the Jaffe response or an enzymatic test. The Jaffe reaction includes forming an alkaline picrate. It is susceptible to both negative (such as bilirubin) and positive blockages (e.g., ketones and proteins). To address some of these difficulties, several changes to the Jaffe reaction have been developed.

BUN
Serum urea/BUN values can also be raised in the presence of a high-protein diet or individuals taking oral corticosteroids.

Protein and urine albumin
Urine albumin and protein may be increased when there are factors other than kidney infection, such as fever, posture, and activity. Furthermore, in the presence of urinary tract pollution, urine protein levels may be elevated in the absence of intrinsic renal disease.

Complications
Complications of most renal capacity tests, aside from those found with venepuncture, are infrequent. GFR estimation with isotopes may be exposed to minimal radiation. However, it is not recommended to have repeated exposures over short periods. A few people may have unfavorable reactions to radiocontrast agents including iodine.

Patient safety and awareness
Patients should be informed about the little quantities of ionizing radiation to which they will be exposed during GFR estimation using

radioactive isotopes. Pregnancy must be ruled out in any female of the childbearing stage before performing this test.

In general, patients who are having blood taken should be warned about the possibility of discomfort and bruising.

Small amounts of preservatives, such as thymol, may be present in 24-hour urine collection containers, and direct contact with the skin and mucous membranes should be avoided. Collection bottles kept away from little children who may inadvertently consume the additives contained inside.

Patients should also be advised to continue taking their usual hydration intake before these examinations.

Chapter 11: Liver Function Tests

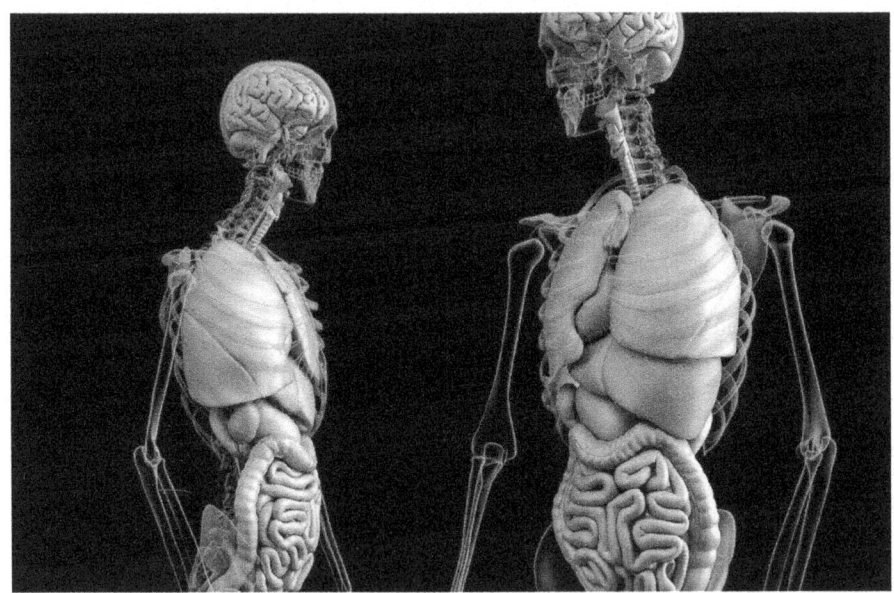

What Exactly Are Liver Function Tests?

Liver function tests, often known as liver chemistries, estimate the amounts of proteins, liver bilirubin, and enzymes in your blood to assist evaluate the strength of your liver.

A liver function test is frequently recommended in the following situations:

- To detect damage caused by liver contaminations such as hepatitis B and hepatitis C.
- To track the symptoms of particular medicines known to harm the liver.
- If you already have a liver infection, monitor the illness and how well a particular therapy is working.
- If you are suffering symptoms of a liver problem.

- If you have certain medical conditions, such as excessive triglycerides, hypertension, diabetes, or weakness.
- If you drink a lot of booze.
- If you have gallbladder disease.

The liver can be subjected to a variety of tests. Certain tests can represent different aspects of liver capacity.

The following tests are often used to detect liver abnormalities:

- Alanine transaminase is an enzyme that converts alanine to alanine (ALT).
- Alkaline phosphatase is a kind of enzyme that breaks down alkaline phosphatase (ALP).
- Albumin.
- Aspartate aminotransferase is a kind of enzyme that converts aspartate to aspartate (AST).
- Bilirubin.

The ALT and AST tests assess enzymes released by your liver as a result of illness or injury. The albumin test measures how efficiently the liver produces albumin, whereas the bilirubin test measures how well it eliminates bilirubin. ALP can be used to evaluate the liver's bile duct system.

Having abnormal findings on any of these liver tests usually requires further investigation to discover the cause of the abnormalities. Even modestly elevated findings might be linked to a liver illness. These enzymes, on the other hand, can be found in locations other than the liver.

Discuss the findings of your liver function test with your doctor and what they may signify for you.

Which of the Following Are the Most Prevalent Liver Function Tests?

Liver function tests are used to measure the levels of certain proteins and enzymes in your blood.

Depending on the test, greater or lower-than-normal amounts of certain proteins or enzymes might indicate a problem with your liver.

Regular liver function testing includes the following:

Alanine transaminase (ALT) test

Your body uses alanine transaminase (ALT) to metabolize protein. If the liver is injured or not functioning properly, ALT can be released into the bloodstream. As a result, ALT levels rise.

A higher than normal score on this test may indicate liver injury.

According to the American College of Gastroenterology, ALT levels of more than 25 IU/L (global units per liter) for women and 33 IU/L for men usually require additional examination and testing.

Aspartate aminotransferase (AST) test

Aspartate aminotransferase (AST) is a molecule present in the heart, muscles, and liver. Because AST levels aren't as specific for liver damage as ALT, they're usually calculated in conjunction with ALT to detect liver problems.

When the liver is injured, AST can be released into the circulation. A high AST result may indicate a problem with the muscles or the liver.

In adults, the normal range for AST is up to 40 IU/L, and it may be greater in infants and young children.

Alkaline phosphatase (ALP) test

The enzyme alkaline phosphatase (ALP) is present in your bile ducts, bones, and liver. An ALP test is usually ordered in conjunction with a few other tests.

Significant levels of ALP may indicate a blocked bile duct in the liver, inflammation, or bone disease.

Because their bones are growing, adolescents and youngsters may have elevated ALP levels. Pregnancy can also cause an increase in ALP levels. These levels in adults typically vary from 60 to 120 U/L.

Albumin test

Albumin is a primary protein produced by your liver. It serves a variety of vital physiological activities. **As an example, consider albumin:**

- Prevents fluid from leaking out of your blood vessels.
- Feeds your tissues.
- Carries vitamins, hormones, and other chemicals throughout your body.

An albumin test determines how effectively your liver produces this specific protein. If you get a low score on this test, it may indicate that your liver isn't operating properly.

The normal albumin range is 3.5 to 5.0 grams per deciliter (g/dL). Low albumin levels, on the other hand, can be caused by inadequate nutrition, infection, renal disease, and inflammation.

Bilirubin test

Bilirubin is a byproduct of the destruction of red blood cells. It is typically metabolized by a person's liver where it passes through before being excreted in your feces.

Bilirubin cannot be properly processed by a diseased liver. This causes an unusually high amount of bilirubin in the blood. A high bilirubin level may indicate that the liver isn't operating properly.

The normal range for total bilirubin is 0.1 to 1.2 milligrams per deciliter (mg/dL). Certain acquired illnesses cause elevated bilirubin levels, but the liver function is normal.

What Is the Purpose of a Liver Function Test?

Liver tests can help you evaluate how well your liver is operating. **The liver performs a variety of vital physiological processes, such as:**

- Eliminating impurities from your blood.
- Obtaining vitamins from the foods you consume.
- Vitamin and mineral storage.
- Controlling blood clotting.
- Synthesis of proteins, chemicals, cholesterol, and bile.
- Developing anti-contamination factors.
- Cleansing your blood from germs.
- Removing chemicals that may be harmful to your health.
- Maintaining hormonal balance.
- Controlling blood sugar levels.

Liver problems can render a person incapacitated and even dangerous.

What Are the Signs and Symptoms of a Liver Disease?

The following are symptoms of a liver disorder:

- Weakness.
- Exhaustion or lack of energy.
- Yellowness (yellow skin and eyes).
- Loss of weight.
- Ascites are fluid accumulations in the abdomen.
- Tainted bodily discharge (light stools or dark urine).
- Nausea.
- Vomiting.
- Diarrhea.
- Discomfort in the abdomen.
- Unexplained bruises or bleeding.

If you are experiencing signs of a liver problem, your primary care physician may arrange for a liver function test. The various liver function tests can also detect disease progression or therapy, as well as evaluate the symptoms of certain medications.

Preparing for a Liver Function Test

Your doctor will give you detailed instructions on how to prepare for the blood sample portion of the test.

Certain foods and medications can affect the amounts of these proteins and enzymes in your blood. Your doctor may advise you to avoid specific types of medicines or refrain from eating anything for some time before the test. Make sure to drink enough water before the exam.

You may need to wear a shirt with sleeves that can be easily pulled up to allow blood test collection.

A liver function test is carried out in the following manner:

Your blood may be obtained at an emergency room or a specific testing facility. To guide the examination:

- Before the test, the healthcare practitioner will clean your skin to reduce the possibility that any germs on your skin may cause disease.
- They will most likely wrap a flexible lash around the arm. Your veins will become more visible as a result of this. They'll take blood samples from your arm using a needle.
- Following the draw, the healthcare professional will apply a bandage and gauze to the cut location. At that time, the blood sample will be sent to a laboratory for examination.

The Risks of a Liver Function Test

Blood draws are common procedures that seldom result in severe responses. **However, the risks of administering a blood test include:**

- Hematoma (under-the-skin bleeding).
- Fainting.
- Extreme bruising.
- Infection.

After a liver function test

After the exam, you can usually depart and get on with your business. However, if you feel light-headed or dizzy after the blood draw, you should rest before leaving the testing facility.

These tests may not inform your primary care physician what ailment you have or the extent of any liver damage, but they may help your doctor identify the next phases. Your doctor will call you to report the results or will examine them with you later.

In general, if your findings indicate a problem with your liver function, your primary care physician will review your medications and previous treatment history to assist establish the cause.

If you drink alcohol excessively, you will have to stop drinking. If your primary care physician determines that a medication is causing high liver enzymes, they will advise you to discontinue taking the medication.

Your doctor may decide that they would like to test you for hepatitis, another disease, or infections that might harm your liver. They may also choose to take pictures, such as an ultrasound or CT scan. They may order a liver biopsy to check for fibrosis, fatty liver disease, or other liver disorders.

Chapter 12: Endocrine Function Test

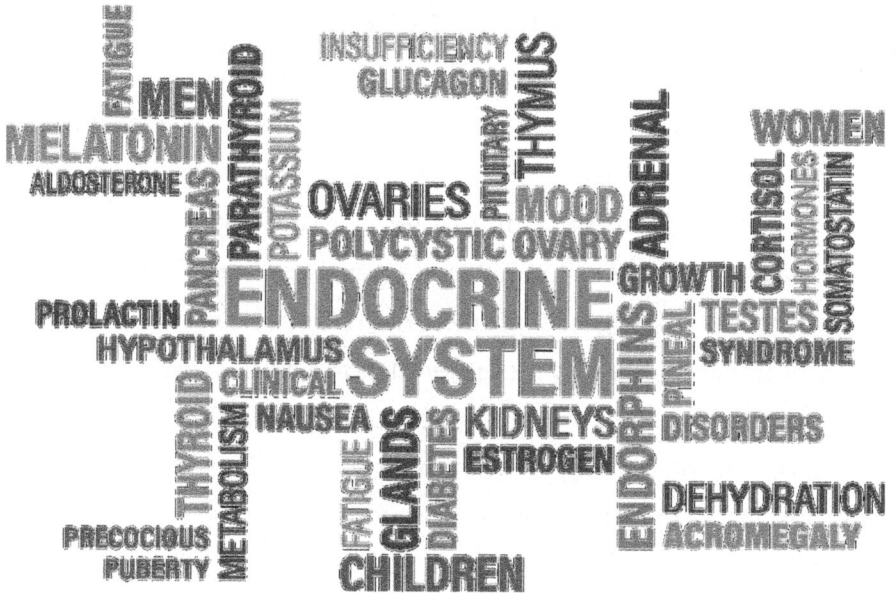

The endocrine system refers to a group of organs that secrete hormones directly into the circulatory system, where they are carried to distant target organs. Most hormones collaborate with the brain and have an indirect or direct influence on each other.

The gonads (ovaries and testicles), hypothalamus (an organ at the base of the brain), pituitary (a gland in the middle of the brain), thyroid gland (under the voicebox), and adrenals (glands located over the kidneys), as well as the liver and pancreas, are the primary glands involved in hormone secretion and activity. Testing for specific hormone levels produced by various hormone-producing glands can identify anomalies that might have a detrimental influence on menstruation and contraceptive function. The endocrine system is critical for reproductive health.

Endocrine Function Fertility Tests

ACTH (adrenocorticotropic hormone)

Excess ACTH can be caused by congenital (present after delivery) adrenal hyperplasia (CAH), which is the expansion of the adrenal glands. CAH is caused by inadequate glucocorticoid production (a class of hormones created by the adrenal gland). In these patients, glucocorticoid precursors accumulate and become androgenic hormones. These androgenic steroids have been linked to infertility. Male hormones produced by the adrenal gland (known as androgens), when present in excess, can cause reproductive problems in humans. Overabundance androgens in women may result in the development of male auxiliary sex traits and the suppression of LH and FSH production by the pituitary gland. Androgen levels may be elevated in women who have polycystic ovaries or a tumor in the adrenal gland, pituitary gland, or ovary. An overabundance of prolactin levels may also be a factor.

Aldosterone

It is a hormone produced by the adrenal glands that control potassium and sodium levels in the blood. More specifically, it aids in the management of blood pressure and the electrolytes and fluids parity in the blood. Measuring the amount of aldosterone released into the body by the adrenal glands can help identify an adrenal tumor, as well as the cause of hypertension or low potassium levels.

C-Peptide

It can serve as a useful indicator of insulin secretion. Low C-peptide levels are typical when insulin production is reduced, as in insulin-dependent diabetes, or suppressed, as in a normal response to exogenous insulin; elevated C-peptide levels may arise from the increased ß-cell activity seen in insulinomas. In the differential diagnosis of hypoglycemia, C-peptide measurement can be used to improve insulin estimates as a file of pancreatic function.

CA-125

It is a protein present on the surface of many ovarian cancer cells as well as a small amount of normal tissue. The test measures the concentration of CA-125 in the blood. It might be used for women who have an ovarian blister, to help identify endometriosis, or follow the endometriosis development.

Cortisol

It is also known as the stress hormone, generated in reaction to stress. Estimation of blood cortisol levels is useful in the differential diagnosis of Addison's and Cushing's disease, adrenal hyperplasia, cancer, and hypopituitarism as an indication of adrenocortical function. Cortisol abnormalities have been discovered in individuals with extreme pain, acute infections, diabetes mellitus, or heart failure, as well as in women who are pregnant or using estrogen therapy.

Growth hormone

This test is typically ordered for individuals who have symptoms of growth hormone anomalies, as a follow-up to other irregular hormone test findings, or to aid in the assessment of pituitary function. The pituitary gland produces growth hormone, which plays an important part in how the body utilizes food for vitality (metabolism). GH is also an insulin antagonist (it blocks insulin and its sugar-lowering effects), which might result in elevated blood sugar levels and diabetes mellitus in sensitive individuals.

Insulin

It is also known as Growth Factor Binding Protein 1 (IGFBP-1) —high insulin levels (hyperinsulinemia) suppress IGFBP-1 production, increasing free IGF-1. IGF-1 works with insulin to increase hyperandrogenism (male hormone overproduction) by increasing testosterone production in the ovaries. As a result, a combination of hyperinsulinemia, elevated free IGF-1, and androgens observed when IGFBP-1 levels are low likely contribute to the endometrial dysfunction, increased miscarriage rate, infertility, and endometrial hyperplasia seen in PCOS.

T3 (Triiodothyronine)

It is a blood test used to assess thyroid function. Ovulation may be influenced by thyroid issues. T3 values clearly distinguish between normal and hyperthyroid individuals (excess thyroid hormone production), since they are elevated in the latter. Thyrotoxicosis might be caused by unusually high levels of T3 instead of T4. Serum T4 (Thyroxin), Thyroxine Binding Globulin, Thyroid Stimulating Hormone, and other clinical findings are also used to assess a person's thyroid function.

T4 (Thyroxine)

It is a blood test used to assess pituitary and thyroid function. Ovulation may be influenced by thyroid issues. T4 (or Thyroxin) is a central thyroid hormone that is largely linked to other (transporter) proteins, the most important of which is Thyroxine-Binding globulin (TBG). Hyperthyroidism (excess thyroid hormone production) is characterized by an elevated level of T4 in the presence of normal amounts of Thyroid-Binding proteins. T4 levels are lower in hypothyroidism (too little thyroid hormone production). In any event, irregular TBG levels may have an impact on the total T4 concentration's ability to detect thyroid health (either hypothyroidism or hyperthyroidism). A T3 Uptake test may be used to determine the degree of TBG involved. When thyroid function is disrupted, the total T4 and T3 take-up quality will be high or low. In normal thyroid patients with abnormal TBG levels, the total T4 and T3 uptake will be distorted in inverse ways (one will be high and the other low or the other way around). The Free Thyroxine Index (FTI or T7), a commonly used measure of thyroid health, is the sum of the T4 and T3 Uptake values divided by 100.

TSH (Thyroid-stimulating hormone)

It stimulates the thyroid organ and causes it to produce T4 and T3. TSH estimation is mostly used to diagnose the cause of hypothyroidism (too minimal thyroid creation). TSH levels are elevated in essential hypothyroidism due to the inability of thyroid hormones to be produced. Thyroid hormone production is reduced in auxiliary or tertiary hyperthyroidism due to pituitary or hypothalamic damage. TSH levels are frequently reduced to subnormal levels in hyperthyroidism (excess thyroid production). TSH can also be used to evaluate whether a patient has enough T4 levels.

Thyroid Peroxidase Antibody (TPO Ab)

It detects autoantibodies directed against thyroid peroxidase (TPO), an enzyme in the thyroid gland, essential for thyroid hormones production. Thyroid peroxidase autoantibodies are produced by the body. TPOAb has the potential to target the thyroid and impair thyroid function. A positive test for these antibodies before starting reproductive therapy indicates an increased risk of miscarriage.

Vitamin D 25 OH

The most precise percentage of vitamin D in the body. Low 25-hydroxy vitamin D levels indicate a vitamin D deficiency, which may result in low blood calcium levels (hypocalcemia), weak or powerless bones (osteomalacia and osteoporosis), and elevated levels of parathyroid hormone (auxiliary hyperparathyroidism). Vitamin D is also linked to infertility since it promotes estrogen production in humans. Inadequate D levels have also been linked to an increased risk of pre-eclampsia (hypertension that develops in certain ladies during the last 50% of pregnancy).

Chapter 13: Miscellaneous Diagnostic Tests

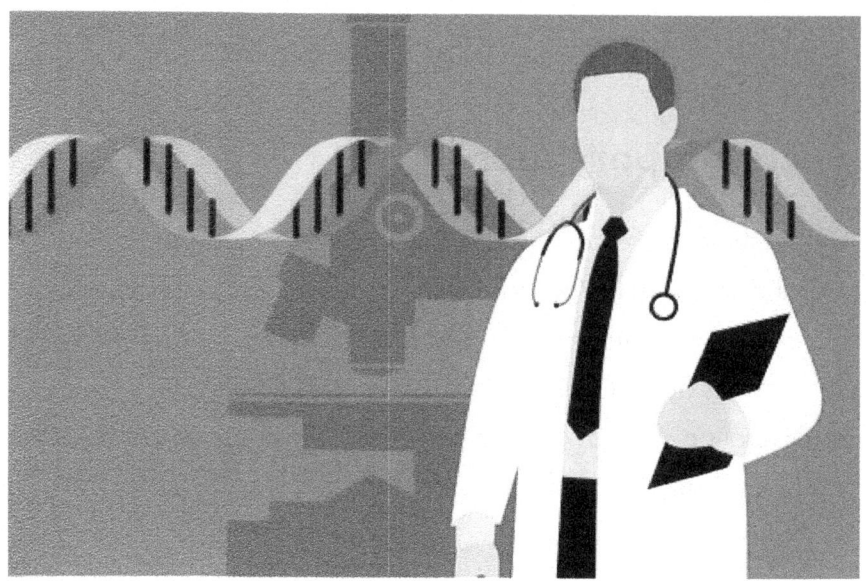

Skin Prick Tests

These may be beneficial in identifying particular allergens that cause IgE-mediated responses. They may have an impact on management and serve as a guide for allergy avoidance. They are also utilized to help determine the existence of atopy. Contact urticaria, atopic eczema, and probable food allergy triggers may also be detected. When compared to a RAST test for a particular IgE, the findings are available nearly instantly and correspond well with RAST test results. They should be performed by personnel who have been trained to read the tests and treat adverse responses.

Common aeroallergens, such as pollens (grass, tree, weeds), molds (Alternaria alternata, Aspergillus fumigatus, Cladosporium, Penicillium chrysogenum), house dust mites (Dermatophagoides pteronyssinus), and animal dander, should be recognized from the history (dog epithelium, cat pelt).

Aspects of Application

- Antihistamines (7 days) and omalizumab (6 months) should be discontinued before testing. The response may also be inhibited by tricyclic antidepressants and phenothiazines. Oral steroids do not appear to suppress test findings.
- There is a very low chance of anaphylaxis; adrenaline and resuscitation equipment should be readily available. Food and latex testing require extra caution.
- Cleanse the skin with a 70% alcohol solution. Apply an allergen drop to the skin (usually on the forearm's inside). A variety of allergies are commercially accessible. For suspected fruit and vegetable sensitivities, using fresh produce.
- Using a needle, prick the skin through the allergen drop (do not draw blood). This should be done using a calibrated lancet (1mm) held vertically or a hypodermic needle at a 45° angle to the skin.
- Histamine is generally the positive control, while the diluent is the negative control (usually glycerinated saline).
- After 10 minutes, check the histamine control, and after 15 to 20 minutes, check the allergen extracts. An itchy weal is a good outcome that should be compared to controls, since some people react only to the skin prick (dermatographism).

- Various test solutions are standardized to provide a mean weal diameter of 6mm across sensitive participants.
- A weal of 3mm or greater is regarded positive (indicating sensitization).
- A positive test result does not indicate that clinical symptoms are caused by bronchial hyperresponsiveness to the tested allergen but raises clinical suspicion. Positive findings can occur in people who do not have symptoms, and false negatives can occur.

Rast

Radioallergosorbent blood tests are more specific than skin prick tests, but less sensitive and costlier and provide comparable results. There is no danger of anaphylaxis, and the patient does not need to cease taking antihistamines before the test.

Unconventional Tests

Electrodermal allergy testing (using a Vega test machine) was created as a supplement to homeopathic prescription and is now extensively used in alternative medicine to determine allergic status to food and environmental allergens. It is based on tiny changes in electrical impedance of the skin at acupuncture sites in reaction to allergens put in an electrical circuit. There are no RCT data to indicate that this technique can distinguish atopic patients from non-atopic persons based on skin prick testing.

Induced Sputum Technique

- It is used to look for infection (e.g., tuberculosis, PCP) or airway inflammation.
- Patients should rinse their mouths and brush their teeth to reduce oral contamination. To reduce bronchoconstriction, use inhaled salbutamol.
- A face mask is used to deliver nebulized hypertonic (2.7 to 5%) saline. Following that, the patient expectorated sputum into a sterile pot.
- If infection transmission (e.g., tuberculosis) is possible, do the test in a negative pressure room with adequate personnel and other patient safety. Do not perform in an open ward or in the outpatient department.
- Send sputum to microbiology as soon as possible for staining and culture, as well as direct immunofluorescent testing for Pneumocystis jirovecii (if indicated). Sputum is combined with 0.1% dithiothreitol, diluted with saline, filtered, and centrifuged to obtain differential cell counts.

Bronchoprovocation Test

Several approaches, including pharmacological challenges (non-specific bronchoprovocation tests), exercise challenge (for exercise-induced asthma), food additive challenge, and antigen challenge, can be used to detect bronchial hyperreactivity.

Non-specific bronchoprovocation test

- Useful if there is a diagnostic uncertainty about the diagnosis of asthma.

- Typically, inhaled methacholine or mannitol are used. Methacholine induces smooth muscle contraction directly. Mannitol is more selective but less sensitive since it operates indirectly through the release of endogenous mediators.
- It should be carried out by skilled people who are equipped to deal with acute bronchospasm.
- Patients must discontinue their normal asthma medication (inhaled/oral steroids for 2 to 3 weeks; antihistamines for 3 days; tiotropium for 1 week; LABA for 2 days).
- Provocation agent dosages are increased progressively, with FEV1 assessed after each dose.

Methacholine is a kind of amino acid. Inhaled using a nebulizer with solutions ranging from 0.03 mg/mL to 16 mg/ml. The test is terminated if FEV1 falls by 20% or the maximum dosage of methacholine is administered. Medication concentration that causes a 20% drop is known as the PC20, and it may be found between the concentrations of the previous 2 doses. A PC20 of 8 mg/mL indicates asthma. PC20 levels in healthy people are greater than 16mg/mL. Patients with a family history of asthma, COPD, or CF, as well as those recovering from viral infections, may have intermediate reactions.

Mannitol's proprietary dry powder inhaler (Aridol®) was employed. A provocation dosage that causes a 15% decrease in FEV1 (PD15) is observed. PD15 indicated asthma at a cumulative dosage of 635 mg.

Cardiac Enzymes Discussion

The primary aim of the study of these enzymes is to help in the diagnosis of MI. However, as you can see from the description of each enzyme, the diagnosis cannot be established fast. The fact that the enzymes are not only found in the heart muscle complicates the diagnosis. The IM injection is one of the most prevalent causes of enzyme increase in the therapeutic environment. The injection will cause muscular damage. Alcohol use and trauma may also produce increases, clouding the diagnosis.

In recent years, isoenzyme test methods have become more sophisticated. Improved measurement and reporting procedures have increased the physician's confidence in the diagnosis. In addition, the MD must rely on additional evidence to make the diagnosis. Polymorphonuclear leukocytosis occurs within 12 to 24 hours after an acute MI event. In some situations, there is also a small elevation in body temperature and a little increase in blood flow rate. When all of the foregoing information is gathered, a MI may be suspected.

The attentive nurse may learn a lot about the patient. She understands the test method(s) utilized to quantify enzymes and isoenzymes at your facility. Some laboratories now display the findings on a very sophisticated laboratory sheet on a graph that visually depicts normal and abnormal results and essentially diagnoses the issue for you.

Test: Myoglobin

This is a blood chemistry test that determines the concentration of this enzyme in the blood. This enzyme is not classified as a cardiac enzyme.

However, myoglobin is frequently utilized to validate the results of cardiac enzymes and confirm the myocardial injury.

Normal Values: 30 to 90 NG/ml

Clinical implications

This test examines myoglobin levels in the blood, which is an oxygen-binding muscle protein comparable to hemoglobin. Myoglobin is present in skeletal and cardiac muscle; it is also released into the circulation following muscle damage. As a result, serum myoglobin levels help estimate the extent of muscle injury. However, because myoglobin does not reveal the location of the injury, it is only used to CONFIRM the results of other tests such as CPK, CPK-MB, and others. Test results must also be compared to the patient's indications and symptoms.

Collecting blood from a patient who has just had an angina attack or cardioversion is not recommended. Myoglobin levels may rise as a result of cardioversion or angina episodes. Because myoglobin levels do not speak for 4 to 8 hours after a MI, doing this test soon after a MI provides deceptive results. A radioactive scan done within 1 week after the test may have an impact on the findings. Skeletal muscle damage, polymyositis, dermatomyositis, systemic lupus erythematosus, shock, and acute renal failure lead to increased myoglobin levels.

Conclusion

The main objective of this book is to provide accurate and straightforward information while also making understanding lab values simple for all readers. This book was designed as a guide to give vital help throughout one's career (student or professional), also for those taking examinations. This book simplifies learning and directs readers' attention to the most significant features of laboratory tests ordered in the hospital.

The findings of clinical laboratory tests are critical in the diagnostic, monitoring, and screening process. More laboratory tests are being sought as the basis for diagnostic decisions. As a result, a large amount of information is made available, making it critical that doctors are well-versed in the tests and how to interpret the results for their patients. To comprehend the laboratory test results, one needs to have a frame of reference that distinguishes between "health" and "illness." As a result, the physician must consider biological variance while interpreting the results and avoid misinterpretation. The impact of random and systematic mistakes on the results and diagnostic sensitivity and specificity are equally important considerations. This book makes it easy for all the professionals and, at some points, for patients to interpret their results.

As professionals, we must keep in mind that our patients are humans just like us. These people present their perspectives, fears, and concerns about the diagnostic procedure and what their disease means to them and their dear ones, what coping methods they employ, what resources are accessible to them, and what additional knowledge they have about themselves. As physicians and healthcare practitioners, we must be willing to "put ourselves in the shoes" of others, that is, to identify with and empathize with the patient's point of view as much as feasible. When we reach that stage, we may begin to understand and interact with one other on the deeper levels required for a therapeutic relationship to develop.

Made in the USA
Las Vegas, NV
05 August 2022